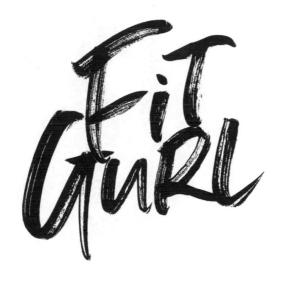

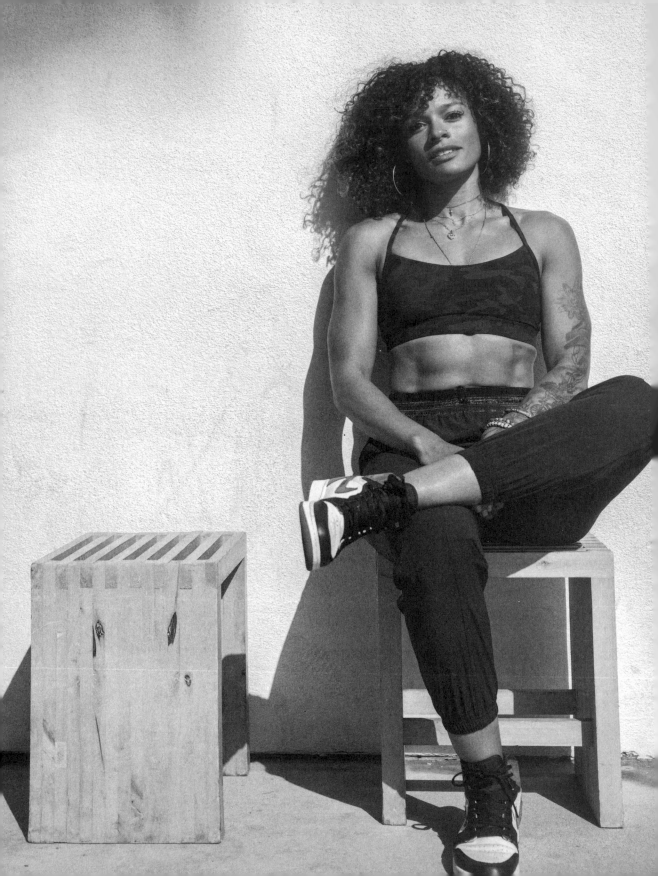

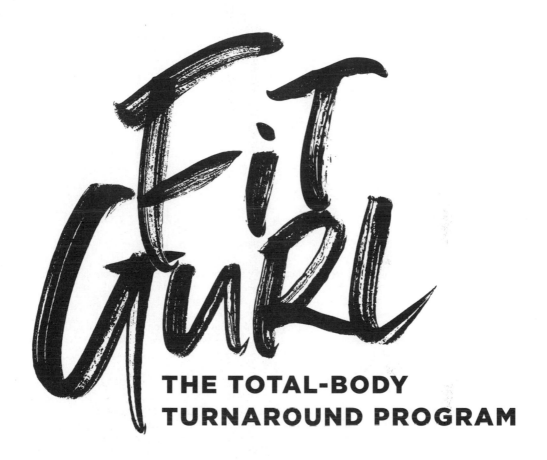

THE TOTAL-BODY
TURNAROUND PROGRAM

Melissa Alcantara

FOREWORD BY KIM KARDASHIAN WEST

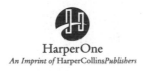

HarperOne

An Imprint of HarperCollinsPublishers

For Victor and Bella

HarperOne

HarperCollins books may be purchased for educational, business, or sales promotional use. For information, please email the Special Markets Department at SPsales@harpercollins.com.

FIRST EDITION

Designed by Matchbook Digital/Kris Tobiassen
Lifestyle photography by Jeff Chu
"Before" photography courtesy of the author
Exercise photography courtesy of Fitplan

Library of Congress Cataloging-in-Publication Data has been applied for.

ISBN 978-0-06-295948-5

20 21 22 23 24   WOR   10 9 8 7 6 5 4 3 2 1

Contents

Foreword by Kim Kardashian West vii

Introduction 1

Part One The Trouble and the Truth

Chapter One | F*ck, I'm Fat!.. 11

Chapter Two | Get Out the Way.. 23

Chapter Three | The Four C's That Will Set You Free:
Control, Connection, Concentration, and Consistency 35

Part Two The Turnaround

Chapter Four | 45°.. 55

Chapter Five | 90° 93

Chapter Six | 180° 117

Conclusion 139

The Turnaround Toolbox

Recipes 143

Exercise Database 197

Foreword
by Kim Kardashian West

A few years ago, I was up in the middle of the night and I was thinking, *I just need to get it together*. I need to figure out what's going on with my body. I need to find someone who cares, who is willing to get up at any hour, someone who will push me harder than I've ever been pushed before. As I was scrolling through Instagram I randomly came across Melissa's page and immediately thought, *I have to work out with her*. It was like our universes aligned. She was moving to LA that week—and has been my trainer ever since.

I assumed I probably couldn't follow her lifestyle to a T—look at her body—but I could tell she is the kind of person I wanted to have around to push me. I wanted her voice in my head, I wanted her to show me how to do a certain exercise or move a certain way, and I wanted her there to inspire me to keep going. I knew she would be really hard on me. I needed her to share with me the same healthy lifestyle that she was living and has worked for her.

Once I started to work out with her I realized, *This is way harder than I thought it would be*. Melissa *pushed* me.

We work out at 6:00 a.m. every day before the kids wake up. I feel so much better and more energized going into my day after I've completed my workout. Sometimes I'm sleepy in the mornings, and it's difficult for me to get going, but Melissa never complains. We share my goals, and she is always there to help me accomplish them.

Melissa taught me a completely different way in the gym. We still do some cardio but she showed me how you can really transform your body using weights and not be afraid of them.

In this book, Melissa will teach you how to care for your body, your health and fitness. Even if you only have a little bit of time to work out and even with limited or no access to a gym, Melissa will help you find a way.

KIM

Introduction

So, since this is an introduction, I thought I'd be super literal about it and introduce myself to you, like a proper person. My name is Melissa Alcantara (pronounced Al-Can-Tar-A) and I'm a personal trainer, mom, and fucking superhero. I grew up in the Bronx, New York, but I spend most of my time now in and around Los Angeles, California. On most days, you can find me in the gym, getting my own workouts in, then at the gym training my clients, then spending time with my daughter or friends. On most days, you can also find me in disbelief that I'm living the life I'm living.

Why? Because I grew up without present parents (like, they were physically never around). I never had any thoughts about what I was going to be or had any real sense of direction. I didn't have a support system or someone to tell me "good job" or help me with homework or put me in a sport. I definitely never felt like I was good enough to be anybody or become someone.

But then something happened to me that changed my life. I mean literally changed the trajectory of my entire life. You're going to think I'm crazy when I say it, but it's 100% the truth. You see, what happened was . . . I started working out.

I know, I know, it sounds ridiculous, and it seems like a super convenient way to introduce my book about health and fitness. But my life honestly changed the day I made my first *real* commitment to do the work to create the body I wanted. That day was seven years ago. I was in my kitchen, and the workout I did made me scream and cry and wince in pain. I thought I might die.

I didn't die. Instead, as it turns out, I actually cracked open the door to my future that day—just the slightest, tiniest hair of a crack, but it was open. Of course, I had no idea. I was just trying to stay alive as Shaun T shouted at me from the TV while I did his Insanity program. I thought for sure I had accidentally stumbled on the workouts designed for professional athletes. *No way* this was a beginner program. (It was.)

I didn't know then that this first workout would lead to dozens more kitchen workouts, which led to me losing 40 pounds, which led to me gaining my confidence and empowerment. And this was all happening as Instagram was becoming more popular, and I remember thinking that I wanted to start sharing more of my story. (This was way before actual "stories" on IG.) Just because my body had changed, and so much of my *self* had changed—I had confidence for the first time ever, I was more in control of my life, I could do anything, I felt I was capable of literally anything—I felt this desire to put it out there in the world. I posted pictures because I wanted to show people that if you put your mind to something, it can be done.

I shared and bared it all: shots of my first attempts at eating healthy, my busted basement gym (at least it was a step up from the kitchen), sweaty post-workout pics, shots of me trying jujitsu or riding around on my bike (it's crazy how gifting yourself with fitness opens up your world to so much!), my "before" pics, my "before booty"—hello, flat butt, no-muscle legs—then my "after" pics, which were all just "in-progress" pics. You know, I put it *all* up on the 'Gram because in addition to the body and the self-growth and the loving myself for the first time, the real gift was sharing my journey and helping people who wanted the same change.

And that's when the craziest thing of all happened. Straight-out-of-a-movie crazy. I got a message from someone saying they worked for Kim Kardashian West and she wanted to know if I might be willing to train her.

I'm sorry . . . WHAAAAAT?! WHOOO? WHAAAAAAAT??!!!

I thought it was complete bullshit at first. Turns out it was the real deal. This chick really worked for Kim Kardashian West and Kim really wanted to meet me. Seriously. Can you imagine that happening out of the blue? I'm pretty sure the odds of me getting hit by lightning in my lifetime were greater than for this to happen.

So, I stepped up my own training a few (thousand) notches, and I started training one of the best known personalities in the world. And it all started with that crazy hard workout, in my crazy tiny kitchen in Brooklyn.

I know what you're thinking: What does this have to do with me? Well, I'm glad you asked. This entire book is for you and about you. I just felt like you had to see at least a snapshot of my experience, so that when I said with The Turnaround anything is possible, you would believe me at least the tiniest bit. Did you get it, that tiniest little bit of belief? Good, because that belief is for *you*, not me. It's for you and the door we're about to open to your future—the one that's out there undiscovered and full of wild and unpredictable possibility.

"START HERE"

I was 28 when I decided I was really ready and willing to make a change in my life. At that point I was a mom who still had a postpartum body over a year after giving birth to my daughter, Bella. (Nothing wrong with a postpartum body . . . but my *pre*-partum was more partying and puffing on cigarettes than any kind of exercising and eating well. So, it wasn't pretty before, and it was even less pretty after.) This was me around that time. ——————→

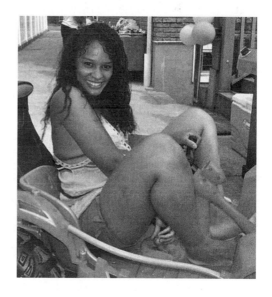

In case you can't tell, this is what a never-been-fit newbie looks like. This was my starting point. I'm sharing this in case you're reading through this introduction and you're on the fence about this program or your abilities, or you are feeling a rising sense of self-doubt—just stop. You now have visual proof that everyone is a beginner at some point.

A lot of the people I meet or who reach out to me on IG say they have all kinds of obstacles to getting fit, as though it's some kind of acceptable reason to not get started. They say it with shame or embarrassment, as though there's something wrong with being at the start of something. I didn't come out of my mother's body with abs! You know what I say to these things? SO WHAT!

So you're a mom . . . to a 3-year-old, a 13-year-old, or a 25-year-old.

So you're 200 pounds.

So you have a 9-to-whenever-they-feel-like-letting-you-go job.

So you don't know anything about fitness.

So you never played a sport.

So you don't know what eating healthy means.

So you're almost 30 or 40 or 50 and you've done maybe 10 jumping jacks in your entire life.

So since you were young you were treated like you were shit.

So . . .

So . . .

So fucking what?!

(*Trigger warning: I like the F word—a lot!*)

All it takes for you to overcome every one of these so-called obstacles is to make the decision that you are committed to making a change in your life. *I* decided. You too can decide these obstacles are just self-doubt masquerading as excuses. You can wake up to the fact that your doubt is wrapped around the feeling that you're not being the best version of yourself. In fact, doubt's grip is so tight you can barely bring yourself to acknowledge the vastness of your untapped potential.

At least that's how it was for me—I was a small planet of self-doubt. Of course, when I first started working out, I couldn't see that this was a big part of what was in my way. I just somehow found a way to override the mess in my head by starting to do the work. And it turns out that the work, no matter how imperfect, is what kills your doubts and in their place leaves space for this amazing thing called confidence. When you start investing in yourself, you give your confidence permission to come alive. And confidence is a practice; you don't just have it, you put in the work and, just like a muscle, it grows.

THE SECRET TO SUCCESS: STOP LOOKING FOR THE SECRET

Everyone always wants a shortcut or hack or *the* trick, that "one thing" that will give them the body they've always wanted. So much of what we see is what we're scrolling through on social media, where everything looks so insta—insta-abs, insta-weight loss. (If you were to just look at my most recent pictures and didn't go back *seven* years, you would have no idea the amount of work I've put in!). But here's the truth: There's no insta-anything. No matter who you are or how much money you have, the real results, the real deal in body transformation, are only achieved through work. That's true of everything in life— so why do we think the body of our dreams should come to us without it?

It's time to get real about this fact, and about what's needed and what's not needed to successfully transform. We are constantly being bombarded with messages trying to convince us we need so much to be successful—protein powders, shoes, headphones, fancy workout pants, other specialized gear, etc.—but guess what? By putting so many things in the way of your progress, you're actually just setting yourself up to fail before you even begin; and you've given yourself something to blame if whatever you try doesn't work.

You don't need *anything* but yourself and your willingness to make a change. There's no fast track or supplement containing the secret to success. Actually, I'll tell you what the secret is—STOP looking for one because it doesn't exist. You get the body you want, the life you want, when you commit to action, you dedicate the time, and you commit to consistency. There are no hacks or shortcuts to success. But there are smarts and strategy . . . which are even better because they'll never fail you.

THE SMARTS AND STRATEGY OF *FIT GURL*

Fit Gurl is not your everyday diet and fitness book (maybe you could tell that already?)—it's a path to self-discovery *through* fitness. As you work out and you get to know your body, maybe for the first time ever, and your body responds in these beautiful, unpredictable ways, you learn to love it and to accept it in a way that's far beyond aesthetic appreciation for things like thin arms, strong legs, or a tight butt. You learn to accept yourself for who you are through this process, and you develop an appreciation for your capabilities that shine through, thanks to work, consistency, commitment. This goes beyond fitness. This is life.

The process doesn't happen with the flip of a switch (remember there's real work involved), but rather in degrees. When we want to right our ship, we've got to turn it around, do a 180. And that's what you're going to discover here in this book—a degree-by-degree shift that redirects you and puts you on the path to your dreams.

You'll discover in the pages ahead a three-part series of rotations designed to turn your life, or at least your fitness, around. (You get what you need from this program!) The rotations will be progressive, from a 45-degree rotation to a 90-degree to a full 180. Then you will be heading in the opposite direction of where you're going now. (Get it? That's your turnaround!) You will learn how to build a body that's fit for life: a strong, ready, and resilient physical form that's mirrored by the same reborn sensibilities in the mind. You will *think* you can do it, and you will be *able* to do it.

Each rotation—45°, 90°, and 180°—will have its own chapter containing eight weeks of "coaching"; 90° and 180° will also each have a free week, which will make the total duration of the program a little over six months. The chapters are structured with a weekly calendar, which will offer daily guidance in the categories of Mouth (food), Mind (mental), and Muscle (the workouts). The sections will each have a distinct focus:

MOUTH: Here you will learn about the area that delivers the most bang for your buck in terms of getting fit: food. I think you'll be pretty stoked to discover the focus on real foods (and plenty of it), not diet foods—nobody can live long term on a diet. Everything you eat will be selected to deliver maximum nutrition. Your goal is not to avoid calories, but to avoid empty calories or calories without purpose. Be prepared to experience a palate change, and to discover simple ways to get more enjoyment out of fresh foods.

MIND: I coach that mental strength comes before physical strength; you must remind the mind what it feels like to do things consistently that create change. While the program on the surface may look like a series of activities geared toward changing the body, they are really changing the mind first. But the mind is not some lump of clay that you just mold into shape and call it a day; it's a nonstop chatterbox that'll pepper you with questions, doubts, and fears like it's got nothing better to do. This is why the "MIND" section in each program chapter will address the evolving voice in your head, and help you feel okay about the kinds of thoughts that come up during your transformation (yes, they're completely normal).

MUSCLE: I don't teach people how to "work out"—I teach them how to TRAIN. Put simply, lifting a weight up and down and jumping side to side is a good workout, but there's no intention, no presence, and thus no real lasting results. My goal is to bring your awareness to your body and help you understand its functioning as a kinetic machine. When you're moving, you should be aware of where everything is, from your toes to your eyes, and seek to control your entire movement pattern. This level of awareness translates to stronger, prettier, and more flexible muscles that you can better use . . . cuz you know where they are, how they feel, and what they're doing.

Everything that's in this program is drawn from my own personal experience: the thoughts that trapped me, the fear of failure, the struggles being honest with myself, the foods I love, the workouts I used to build my body (the one that's so much better than the one I thought I wanted—better because it's stronger and so much more capable than I ever could have imagined). I'm sharing it all with you because it's what I learned through my own process. It's straightforward as shit, and sometimes I may come at you in a way that makes you uncomfortable—but you deserve the honesty. Knowing and understanding what real transformation can feel like will make you that much more durable and diligent in forging your own path.

I'm so glad you are here. For real. You are in for the surprise of your life. When you complete The Turnaround, the discovery of your secret strengths, your unexpected weaknesses, and the whole bundle of unpredictable intimate revelations of who you are and who you can be when challenged will reveal something greater than you could ever have imagined: a degree of self-love and acceptance that you will connect to and hold on tight to through this one awesome life you get to live. (Okay, it might help a little that you're doing it with the ass of your dreams . . .)

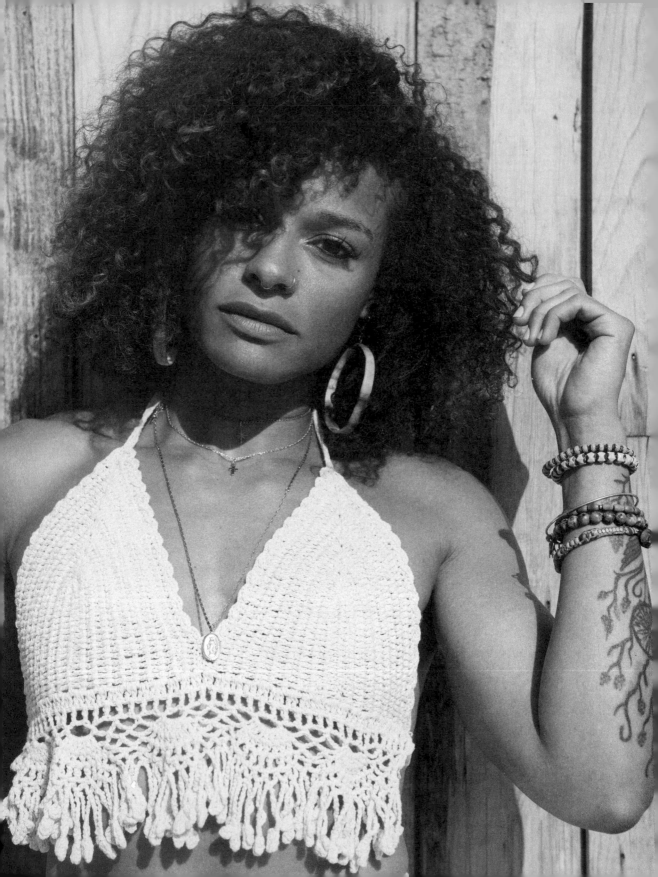

Part One
The Trouble and the Truth

Chapter One

F*ck, I'm Fat!

Oh my God—is this my body forever?
—26-YEAR-OLD ME

I had come home from the hospital with my brand-new baby, Isabella Mia Alcantara, aka punchine, cutie pie, chabelliiii, and huney, born July 14, 2011. She was amazing: a gorgeous ball of new life (that I was totally terrified of, if I'm being honest). But she was mine—well, ours—and now that she had escaped my body and was on the outside needing to be cared for, it was me who felt trapped in my body. I looked at myself in the mirror and wondered aloud if it would be this way forever.

Fast-forward one year . . .

I cannot believe my body still looks like this.
—27-YEAR-OLD ME

The first year of Bella's life seemed to swallow me up. Being a mom is wild, better than I ever could have imagined, but damn, it's hard-ass work being a parent. I was so busy taking care of my new baby, trying to figure out the whole breastfeeding thing, checking to see if she was still breathing every five seconds—if I could make it that long—that I could not make time to do anything else. I couldn't dedicate time to eating healthy and losing weight. (But I could, curiously, make plenty of time to eat or get crappy food. Funny how that works, isn't it?)

I had severe postpartum depression, so when I think back on this time, I try not to do it with blame or shame or self-criticism. I don't know that I could have done better than I did. I didn't feel my best, I certainly didn't look my best, but I was *doing* my damn best to get through each day with one baby Bella still healthy and vibrant and one momma Mel still standing.

Most calm moments were dedicated to eating everything I could get my hands on, and I couldn't stop myself no matter how hard I tried. Or in reality, how hard I *thought* about trying. If thinking about trying was a sport, I no doubt won the gold medal.

As my new life became my new normal and my real post-baby body—that's the one that was 25 pounds lighter after the liquids, the baby, and the inflammation were gone—showed up and was still 170 pounds, those thoughts really started to run rampant, doing double-back layouts, full twists across the mat of my mind. I was nonstop dedicated to the sport of thinking about wanting my body back, but not really doing anything about it. Can you relate?

By the way, this would probably be a good time to make something super clear: This is by no means a "mom's only" sport. Girls, women, ladies, gals, chicks, chicas across the globe are good at the Game of Groans—you know that series produced, directed, and acted by you where you constantly binge-watch the episodes of you beating yourself up, whining, objecting, over and over again, all while taking *zero* action to change—good show, isn't it?! *Highly* recommend it. All it takes is a lot of action in your mind, a lot of inaction in your body, and a poor-me pity party combined and stuck on repeat. If you've spent a lot of time thinking about something you want so bad, and you've done nothing to actually make it happen but sit your ass on your couch and feel sorry for yourself then you can relate. No baby required!

What's funny, or not-so-funny, I suppose, is that this mental "exercise" is so counter-productive. You're literally not doing anything that will get you what you want, but then you're whining (is it still whining even if it only happens in your head and no one else hears it? You bet your ass it is) about it like there's some grand sort of unfairness taking place, a scheme against you occurring on the outside. That's how I felt, at least. I started to feel mad at the world for not giving me the answers or for not making me thin or for not making me feel beautiful. *Why the hell does this have to be so freaking hard? I have to actually do the work, you mean like I have to go out there and figure it out and do stuff? For fuck's sake.*

That kind of anger at others, at whatever external forces you've decided aren't fulfilling your dreams for you, is toxic shit. You might think it's harmless, but left simmering it'll bubble up into resentment and spill over onto your spirit and eat away at your ability to love others and even yourself. I know that might sound a little too self-helpy, but it's true—it's all about you, babe. And by that, I mean if you want to get the body you've always wanted, you are the only one who can do it. Your sweat. Your tears. Your curls— biceps, that is. Your stanky piles of workout clothes. Your gritting teeth. Your winking at yourself in the mirror at the gym. Your shoulders burning, your quads shaking, your fat melting, your muscles shimmering, your smile beaming when you surpass a goal, your smokin'-hot ass turning heads, your confidence busting out of your bright face when you build yourself up and into the person you want to be.

Okay, whoa—are you still there or are you already at the gym working out? I got a little pumped up for a minute and should back it up a bit. My point in all this is to say that there is a "before" headspace just as much as there is a "before" body. I just want you to be aware of this, and maybe start in this first chapter of the book to think about the thoughts that run your world, and how they're contributing to creating your reality.

For me, I didn't even realize the mental loop in which I was stuck until I started looking back at the beginning of my own turnaround, my own transformation. And I sure as hell didn't realize that if you were to fast-forward a few years from those days when I was a new mom crunching on Cheetos on the couch and complaining about the state of my body, you would see me in a gym training Kim Kardashian West, yelling at her to get her butt to the ground when she does squats. Or that I would be getting a hug from Dwayne "The Rock" Johnson after one of the most intense and grueling experiences of my entire life on his show *The Titan Games*. It's no exaggeration to say that I wouldn't have believed you in a million years if you told me either of those experiences would be in my future.

Honestly, it's still so far-fetched to me that this was my future—even though it has all actually happened—I kind of still feel like I'm dreaming. It's just that my life didn't seem to have that kind of trajectory. But once you start The Turnaround you never know where it will take you. It all starts with waking the fuck up.

THE WAKE-UP

"I don't want to feel like this anymore." I was so tired of looking at myself in the mirror and seeing the reflection of my very own decisions; I was tired of playing the lead in "Poor-Me Mel," also written and directed by *me*! No more.

Something in me had had enough; I was at the end of my rope. Are you at the end of your rope? You know you're there when there's no doubt in your mind (fears about the unknown maybe, but no *doubt*) that you are ready to change, and there are no excuses that would be good enough this time.

Before, I would have accepted the excuse that I didn't have everything (I thought) I needed, or I would have questioned my decision about where to start or felt defeated by the lack of clarity in my plan. But something was different this time. This time, I had only the littlest bit of information to start with, and I felt like goddamn Goldilocks—it was the "just right" amount of information. You know why? It had nothing to do with the actual information, how good it was, or how much there was of it, and everything to do with the fact that I told myself it was exactly what I needed. Hello, light bulb moment!! And it wasn't just in my head that I had triggered full-blown engagement, it was in my bones, too—I could *feel* that it was really time to make shit happen.

And, in truth, that is the most important element of all: simply telling yourself—until it becomes a deep understanding, a knowing—that you're right where you need to be. The rest you can fill in as you go. You've got to commit to taking full control of your body in the absence of any proof whether or not it's a step in the right direction.

I wanted this change so bad; I *needed* this change. Starting was a struggle because I knew that once I started, I'd have to go all the way—my success, even my life (dramatic, I know, but it seriously felt that way) depended on it; there would be no going back. I couldn't go into things thinking about how I was going to allow myself to cut corners or skip days; I knew I had to go all in.

Another few weeks went by, and though I was not "ready," I told myself I was. I knew that no time was better than now, because NOW is always the best time to start (even right NOOOOOOWWWWW is perfect, too).

I had picked a program based on my current life situation: I was a mom with a job and a baby, so I needed workouts I could do at home—at least to start—and I knew that I had to change my diet, so I chose something that would give me some basic nutrition guidance.

I went into day one ready. I had packed my food the night before: breakfast, lunch, and two snacks. I was optimistic—just one hour into my fitness journey and I already felt accomplished! But there were so many tasty-looking tests still to come. At the time, I was working as a fashion photography producer in Soho, New York City. Every day we had meetings accompanied with cookies, cakes, sandwiches, and sometimes alcohol—talk about needing to resist temptation.

I went into this program aware of these challenges—I knew that I'd be constantly tempted to make choices that would go against what I was trying to achieve for myself. I knew that I needed willpower; I was always just one cookie away from fucking up the good feeling you get when you're making the right choices. You know that feeling, the one you get when you're doing things that are for *you*—not selfish things, but actions that fall in line with your goal. For a lot of us, these actions involve showing ourselves some legit love and care (the kind we typically reserve for other peeps). You feel that shit! And you feel it when you don't do those things, too—that's for damn sure. It was bigger than just resisting "the cookie"; I needed to show myself that I could do something for me and me only, and I needed the mental momentum to build.

That day at work, I timed and ate my meals just right. I didn't know anything about meal timing, but I had a basic sense of structure, and that's all I needed. I got through the day without straying from my plan—this was the first half of my first day the way I envisioned my first day would be. I checked all the boxes—I was so impressed with myself. Then I realized there was one thing I didn't do: the workout! Fuuucckkk. I got off work around 7:00 p.m. and had not worked out at all. But this was normal for me back then because 1) I was making minimum wage, so I needed the hours, and 2) photography production was notorious for requiring ridiculously long hours. If I was going to let this be my excuse today, I was opening the door to it being the excuse every day.

Did I feel like working out? FOOK, NO. Did I do it anyway? FOOK, YES. I spent all day fighting temptations, feeling hungry, thinking about my next meal, eating on time—in the office closet, if I had to! Was that enough to get abs? I looked down at my belly and still no sign of abs. I guess eating right for one whole day doesn't give me the right to fuck it up in the end. So, I got home and got my workout in. Why? Because *this time I wasn't giving up on myself*—that was the whole point. Remember?!

The days following my decision were the most important and would change my life forever. You know why? Because I *woke up*. I woke up to my potential, my power, my ability to make choices that would make fucking progress happen. To make choices that create real changes. Even that first day I was snapped out of my stupor by these silly, small acts that I'm sure no one else gave a damn about. *"You ate a chicken breast and salad instead of a pile of cookies that you washed down with an almond milk Frappuccino—and you went almond because you're on a "diet" and the regular milk one is not diet-friendly, right? Well, good for you, Melissa"* (pats self on back). It wasn't a big deal, but it was the biggest deal to me, as if I had climbed some sort of mini Mount Everest.

EXCUSE ME, HAVE YOU SEEN MY CORE?

If you've ever watched any of my IG stories or video posts, you know that I'm not shy about how I feel during hard-ass workouts—I curse like a sailor, complain, grit my teeth, shout, and maybe even drop a tear or two. But that's okay, I still get that shit done.

Well, let me tell you that even after years of tough workouts, some of the hardest are the ones I did when I was first starting out. It's not just that I was hella weak, it was also that I didn't know about my body. But Shaun T's Insanity was there to introduce me to it! I had picked this program as the first one I would truly commit to, and it was *definitely* insane.

I still remember this part of it that was called the "Insanity Fit Test"—it was literally a test designed to let you know how much you sucked. At least that's how I felt. The Fit Test was a 25-minute test made up of a certain number of moves that would be included in the daily workouts. There were exercises such as suicides (burpees), switch kicks, power jumps, power jacks, power knees, globe jumps, push-up jacks, and low-plank obliques. (At the time, it felt like I was reading a foreign language.) I hated every move in the Fit Test—they were hard as fuck! And you had to do the test every two weeks.

The first time I took the test, I had no idea what to expect of the moves and of myself. But just two minutes into it, I felt like a complete moron who couldn't even move my body. I was already trying to figure out how in the heck I was going to do the program if I couldn't even survive the test meant to gauge your fitness. It was the worst, worst performance of my life. But on the bright side, I can say that it lit a five-alarm fire under me to get it together and get my ass in shape.

The best thing about starting F-A-R down the ladder is that you can only get better. (How much better? That is up to you!) I knew I had eight weeks to get better, and that meant each and every workout I had to do my best in order to make the most out of the commitment I made. I was on a fucking mission.

I wanted to puke, I wanted to cry—I did cry a few times—and I really, really wanted to quit. But the further I got into it, the more consistent I was, I knew that I just couldn't go back because that would mean giving up. There was no way I was going to give up on myself.

I had yet to even pick up a weight. But because I was so out of shape and didn't have any muscles or coordination, I would find myself with little injuries that would almost prevent me from working out the following day. My ankle would hurt, my left knee would ache, my shoulder would feel kind of funky. All this was because I was just throwing my body around and I had no awareness of my body. (The fancy word for this is *proprioception*, but whatever you want to call it, I had noooone of it.) Each workout I would listen to the exercise instructions and watch the people in the video do the moves and just try my best to mimic their form. I'm sure if I had video of myself, it would have looked like the fitness version of Pinterest fails. It didn't matter, though—I was paying attention, and things were changing.

I remember one specific day about four weeks into the program when Shaun T said, "Use your damn core, Melissa." (Okay, maybe it was just "use your core," but it sure seemed like he was talking directly to me.) I think I was doing high knees and I tucked my ass and it was like it finally connected: "Oh shit! My abs are lifting my legs rather than me trying to swing them up"—or something like that. I have this physical recall of the feeling of being able to send a message to my body and my body not only listening but responding in the way it was supposed to. The phone had been ringing and ringing for a long-ass time and someone on the other end finally answered. That's when I knew that this was the beginning of something amazing.

THANK YOU, NEXT . . . LEVEL

After I finished Insanity, I was ready to take it to the next level. I bought just a few weights. Have you ever gone to the supermarket looking for dumbbells? I SURE DID! This was the time before I could afford sweet ol' Amazon Prime to help a woman out. I actually ended up finding a pair of 20-pound Reebok-branded dumbbells on Craigslist—you know I had to get Reebok dumbbells because those *for sure* make you fitter, right?

It was right around this time that I started entering the world of fitness marketing. I was convinced that I needed Nike and brand names that everybody knew to make me fit. I'm sure you have looked at the Insta accounts and, just like me, felt like you couldn't possibly be fit if you didn't have all the things in the photo—because without those leggin's, water bottle, duffle bag, etc., how was I possibly going to get it done?! At least that's what advertisers and influencers want you to think—by buying the look, you will realize and achieve your value. This is utter bullshit, and if you want to talk about bullshit, fear not cuz there's tons of that in the fitness world—and we are for sure gonna talk more about it!

#NoFilter Snapshots of a Real-Deal Beginning

There is so much information available to us these days—seriously, we can find an answer to every question we could ever imagine. And that means you can look up people eating right and working out and find thousands of options, and they'll all just look super fly and shit (except for me—I share the fuckups too!). So, that's great, right? You *want* someone who looks like they know what they're doing showing how it's done. It's great . . . mostly. The problem is that none of these people are just starting out, and that can be more intimidating than it is inspirational.

Let me tell you a little secret: Your beginning can look however the fuck you want it to look. Here are a few "snapshots" of how my beginning looked:

This was me: cotton T-shirt, cotton leggings, and whatever sneakers I could find. No expensive workout gear. No moisture-wicking fabrics or shit like that. Not even a fancy water bottle in sight. Just a glass of plain ol' water straight outta the tap.

This was my gym: Every single day I'd follow the same procedure:

1. Move the kitchen island toward the back window to have enough space to exercise/die.

2. Move everything that was on the kitchen island so that it wouldn't end up on the floor because of the jumping!

3. Set up the old laptop on the kitchen island—usually having to connect the charger to the laptop because the battery would die within 10 minutes.

So, since "Feebok," "Bdidas" and "Nke" were more within Vic's and my price range, I got my weights off Craigslist along with a bunch of retro-era bodybuilding equipment that included: old-ass barbells, plates, a bench, and a solid amount of rust and other people's sweat, dreams, and maybe even someone's blood from a 1980s murder scene. We borrowed a friend's car to drive from Brooklyn to New Jersey to go pick all this stuff up. It took two hours to get there, one spent covering a two-block distance—thank you, NYC traffic! I gave some cash to an old dude in his basement, and back we went another two hours home to Brooklyn. I couldn't have been more excited to lift!

This was who gave a shit: My baby, Bella, would normally be asleep, but sometimes she would wake up and actually join my husband, Vic, and me for the workout. At just over one year old, she could already point to her biceps, quads, abs, and many other muscles! Vic wouldn't believe that I was waking up at 5:00 a.m. to "jump up and down like a crazy person" in our kitchen, and then by week two he was saying, "I'll do the damn workout with you; how hard can it possibly be?!" After nearly puking within the first 10 minutes, he worked out with me every day without missing a single workout.

This was how it all went down: I would pour myself some water and extra water—that way I wouldn't permit myself to take more than the allowed breaks (sometimes you've got to be smarter than yourself to win the game). Then, I would:

- Procrastinate by walking around the house three times.

- Hit Play and then Pause immediately! "Are you ready?" I would ask my hubby like I was waiting on him and not me.

- Pee six times before starting. Flush. Breathe deeply—and pray that I could get through the workout, and then hit Play for real this time.

I was in my own home so that meant I could make whatever noises, look crazy, make faces, breathe loudly, and really push past my limits without judgment. My clothes would also be fully soaked to the point that I could squeeze sweat out of them every day; I had no idea that my body could produce that much sweat.

THE FIRST CHAPTER

Have you ever had a one part coffee, three parts whole milk, with four sugars? That's how you say how much sugar you want at the bodegas in NYC. They make this "coffee" by over-filling a spoon—four times in this case—with sugar and dumping it into your coffee and handing it to you in a blue cup with the words "We Are Happy to Serve You" written on the side. Almost every morning, I would get my coffee this way and have just that and a cigarette for breakfast. For years, too. This is where I come from; this is not who I have to be anymore. This is where I come from—and this is what or who I should feel bad about? Nope.

This is what my body used to look like . . . and this and this and this and all this right here: I should definitely feel bad about this, right? NO freakin' way. It is all part of my story. And I believe 100% that the only way that I was able to start a new chapter in my story was to begin it without throwing shade to all the pages that came before. Your backstory isn't your conclusion, no matter how crappy it is. There might be pages about crappy dietary choices, lazy-ass days, even years, aging, hormonal changes, bigger life stuff like personal traumas, loss, or pain or neglect—man, there are some pages that I want to tear out and burn the fuck up!! But that wouldn't change a thing. It would all still be there, like those damn Whac-A-Moles. All of it has contributed to who you are today, and for better or worse, it has given you the body you have right now. No matter the specifics of your story, it didn't just happen overnight; there're some juicy details behind those juicy thighs.

My point is that I knew things were going to be different for me that day when I started working out. And I want them to be different for you this time ("different" meaning successful). You know why I knew? Because from the very beginning I didn't talk shit about myself. This time I told myself, "You CAN do this!" I was actually behaving like the person I wanted to be. No, I wasn't that person yet, right then and there when I started, but I was making the choices that kept me going in that direction every day. Every decision, every failure, every little bit of success—they were all part of the person I was striving to become. So say it with me: *"I will not talk shit about myself this time. I am not too fat, too weak, too hungry, or too tired. I will achieve what I want to achieve."*

Be mindful of that fucked-up desire to self-sabotage because it is *so much harder to do than to not do.* It's in the space of not doing that we find the first wave of excuses, and then the tsunami of "I'm not good enoughs" starts. Most of us are so twisted that we prefer this negative surge to the risks involved in taking action. Let me tell you, though, pressing Play on that workout on your laptop, lacing up your shoes, getting your kitchen crunches on, laughing at yourself when you realize you were holding the weights wrong—these are opportunities . . .

Who gives a fuck about the past of cigarettes and sugar and the "I can'ts"—which are really "I won'ts"? I'm working to live a new and meaningful life, and for that you can't steal pages from your old script, the one that didn't pan out for you, the one you're trying to leave behind. In order to change the story, I had to become my own number one fan, my biggest supporter, my personal 24/7/365 cheerleader. And you've gotta be that for yourself, too. Nobody else is going to do that for you. Nobody (insert a thousand exclamation points here). The best part of this is realizing that the job of a number one fan is to be crazy encouraging, that there is power in this. You now have the power to say loving things to yourself all day long (you always had it, you just didn't know it was there).

So there's Chapter 1 of *Fit Gurl*. From my heart, mind, soul, and sore-ass muscles straight to yours. (Oh, wait, you haven't done the workouts yet. Just. You. Wait. You'll see what I'm talking 'bout with the muscle . . .) I share my story because I want you to see that there's nothing special about me. I'm just a girl who finally decided to stick with something, to see something through instead of short-changing herself. I saw where I was headed and I thought, *I'm gonna turn this shit around*. And I did. Now, it's your turn.

FIT GURL CHAPTER 1 TO-DO LIST

1. **POSITIVE SELF(IE)-TALK.** Find a picture of yourself you don't like and give yourself a compliment. Not like your awkward-year photos that even your mom would have a hard time complimenting, but you know the one—you probably have a picture of it in your head already! That one where you're at brunch with your friends and you think everyone else looks so fucking perfect and then there's you with your fat arm ruining everything. Or maybe it's the one where someone snapped a pic as you're laughing your ass off and your neck just seems like it didn't get the memo to show up for the picture . . . it's all just chin to chest, and all you can think is *Do I really look like that??* Look at that picture again. Do it. Love it. Love something about yourself with all the real feels.

2. **CHECK YOURSELF.** Are you an excuse hoarder? You know you're one if you seem to always have a reason at the ready for not doing shit: *Ah, I cannnn't* [fill in the blank] . . . *I got this thick-ass hair that takes forever to dry so I'm not going to make it. I'd love to enjoy* [awesome opportunity], *but my little doggie needs its walkie at exactly 6:35 every night or she gets really upset.* Sometimes we get stuck saying things like this without even thinking it through. It's as though we've been programmed and things just jump out of our mouths without real processing. Yet every day and situation is brand new and we can make room in our lives for brand-new answers. I'm not saying that you have to do anything differently just yet. Just start surveying how you respond to opportunities, options, chances, and change. Take notes.

3. *REMEMBER THIS:* **NO ONE STARTS IN THE MIDDLE.** People constantly say things to me like "If I was comfortable lifting weights, I would totally love going to the gym . . ." or "Maybe if I didn't feel so awkward in the gym, I could get into it." Do you understand how absurd that sounds? The reality is that no one starts at the top, let alone in the middle—we all begin at the bottom! Of course, it's natural to want to jump into the center of the groove or to already be in the zone. Nothing in life is like that—why would it be different with your body and fitness? You've got to start in the mucky mess. It's exactly where you're supposed to be.

Chapter Two

Get Out the Way

It's difficult to think of a topic that generates more opinions than health and fitness. You go to the dentist, and the assistant cleaning your teeth might go on and on about keto this and keto that while you're stuck with your mouth wide open and all you can do is nod and say "mmhmm." Your mailman delivers you a fitness magazine and before you know it, he's telling you about how he's really into CrossFit and asking if you've ever tried it. Or the best is when a parent or older relative (no disrespect!) tells you about some really cool fitness tracker that they just put on their phone. "Do you count your steps, too?? You really should."

All I have to say is *DAyyyyum*. Okay, everybody with their PhDs in exercise science issued by Google U needs to CHILL. Because it seems to me that a lot of people are more talk than action—it's more about the TMI and not the BMI, you know what I'm saying?

I don't mean to imply that people aren't legitimately trying diets and exercise methods, or that there's not value in sharing and comparing experiences; there's just way too much noise out there. The onslaught of information and ideas makes it feel nearly impossible to pick a lane and stay in it (which is really all you've got to do to create real change). Consider that a quick Google search for "fitness plan" came back with well over *two billion* results. No joke. We've officially overcomplicated a process that at its foundation is so freakin' simple.

It would be one thing if those two billion results just led you straight to plans you could use—that alone would make it tough enough to choose a starting point. But if you counted all the products being pushed with those plans, you'd have a billion other things being promoted as essential to your fitness or weight loss success: You gotta get this protein powder, dem dope shoes, those fly-ass, expensive-as-shit headphones, those Lulus . . . and you have got to get all of it *before you even start* because it's going to help motivate you and might even just magically melt your pounds away!

Before any of you call me out, saying, "Girl, I know you like your Lulus or Gymshark pants, and Nike and Converse shoes," you bet your ass I love to look and feel a certain way when I work out. That's not my point. My point is that none of it is actually *needed* for success, yours or mine. And it sure as hell isn't necessary for you to get any of this crap before you get started. All these perceived needs can get in the way of your progress because they work as built-in targets of blame if whatever you try doesn't work. This is just the tip of the iceberg of shit we can blame for not achieving what we want with our bodies (and our lives, frankly).

That's what this chapter is about—the iceberg of shit, so much of it submerged below your conscious awareness, that you *allow* to get in the way of achieving your goals. It's all one big fucking head game. And you've got to get a grip on what's going on in your head before you can be successful with The Turnaround.

THE FIRST FAULT

It's pretty obvious where we start with blame—our families, of course. That's where we were formed, by blood or by bond, for better or worse. We were molded by our parents, siblings, grandparents, and whoever else might have contributed to raising us.

The easiest place to point the finger is at your own biological beginning—in other words: your genes. Maybe your mom passed along her pear shape or thick upper arms, your dad his compulsive eating habits or tree-trunk waist. My case was a bit different. I seemed to *not* get the genes that ran in my family. Everyone was basically thin while I was the shy, chunky girl. By shy, I mean having no confidence or self-esteem, and by chunky, I mean being slightly larger everywhere from my feet to my face. I don't know that it would have bothered me that much if it weren't for the fact that I grew up with five other girls—my sister and four cousins—who were all beautiful and thin, and I was constantly comparing myself to them.

My cousins and my sister—the people who were my family and closest to me—also used to say that I was "big" and "rough" and that I wasn't "feminine." This made me feel different and unwanted; I felt that I was invisible. I was the odd one out and I didn't know WHY. This WHY haunted me for so long, but here's the thing: There's no good answer to that WHY, and even if there were an explanation, it wouldn't matter. It would only work to keep you focused on the problem when the solution is really what you seek.

It's possible too that you were raised without being given any clues about how to eat right or get fit. I definitely didn't get any solid health habits passed along to me when I was a kid. My mother worked two or three jobs while my dad was MIA from any parental responsibility.

Don't get me wrong—my mom tried her hardest, between jobs, to keep healthy things around. But the issue was that she had no idea what healthy was herself and got her "health and wellness" advice from Dr. TV.

Things weren't much better in the exercise department either. We didn't have anyone around to ask us what sports or physical activities we were interested in pursuing, let alone take us to practices and games. A weekend trip to the park was our equivalent of finding a unicorn in the wild.

I guess this is what happens when you grow up in the 'hood. Everyone in the neighborhood was pretty much in the same situation you were. I don't even remember seeing people exercising or talking about getting fit, and nobody I knew went to the gym.

You might have had a different upbringing. Maybe you were in one of those mythical families that went to the gym together, or you got to compete in kids' 5Ks or swim on a swim team—and your parents had time to slog you around to these things, and to soccer, basketball, volleyball, whatever-ball games. Good for you. But guess what? You still got that iceberg of shit. I know it. And you know it.

Because later in life, we get to aim those blame bullets at our chosen and created families—our significant others, kids, closest friends, even our co-workers—"That biatch, Sheila, she brought in all those donuts and I *had* to eat them!" If you cohabitate with another human, maybe that person likes crap foods and those foods are always in the kitchen staring at you waiting to be eaten . . . you know those Cheetos with eyes (insert big eyes emoji).

Or perhaps it's the time that other humans demand from you that has the target on it? If you're in charge of getting dinners on the table and doing the laundry, all that thankless stuff that consumes time like a black hole, it's easier to blame any and all of that for missing a workout or for not being able to stick to your plan.

And kids. HOLY SHIT. Talk about demanding. I wouldn't want to be on demand for any other little soul than my daughter and I love her beyond . . . but this is the one area where it can get slippery when it comes to self-care.

Being there for your children is the number one responsibility all parents have. Yet as kids get a little older and the hobbies pile up and their mini-manipulation skills get better, your kids can become all-consuming creatures that all but steal your life from you.

It's the easiest thing in the world to add kid stuff to the iceberg of shit because there's a selflessness to the time and effort you dedicate to your children; it's good for them and it makes us feel good about ourselves. But if you aren't careful, an unrelenting commitment to an absolute prioritization of your kids can resurface as resentments down the road.

I'm not saying that you should be a selfish kind of parent and stop taking your kids to gym classes, birthday parties, and whatever. I'm just telling you that there's a time—it's called when-mama-wants-to-do-something-for-herself time—when you've got to back up and evaluate things. We can get so stuck on creating structure and stability for kids that we forget to ask questions, have conversations, *ask for help*—all things that can open up options that we never knew were there.

You know, maybe try asking yourself things like *Does my kid really need to play three sports, especially when she cries through most of dance class? Is there someone who could handle pickup on the days when I've committed to getting in a workout after work?*

This is the kind of attention and evaluation that needs to happen around *all* the excuses that you allow in your life. You've got to start questioning, even interrogating, their existence. Start problem solving before lack of self-care and self-commitments become bigger problems. We'll come back to this . . .

THE FOOD HABITS OF OTHERS

So, if you're some kind of alien and none of the excuses I've mentioned so far are part of your particular iceberg of shit, how about you try this one on for size: your family- or friend-enforced food habits. This is more than your genes; these are the cultural or social influences around what you put in your mouth each day.

When I was growing up, we didn't have money to buy quality food; we just had food stamps, so we bought whatever we could with that. When we weren't buying government food, we were buying Chinese food. When my mother was home and she had a little time between her jobs, she'd cook and make us rice with beans and chicken. Since she was born and raised in the Dominican Republic, she would cook Dominican food for us, which meant everything was saturated in oil, salt, and butter. Vegetables weren't really a part of our diet and health was never a topic for discussion.

That said, my mom wasn't totally oblivious to diet trends. She would buy things like wheat bread and wheat pasta, and I remember for, like, one second she talked about how we should eat foods that weren't super salty or stop eating "so much sugar." But that didn't change the fact that we were left home alone most of the time, so we ate *whatever* we wanted to eat—every fried, salty, sweet, processed (the more processed the better) food we could get our hands on, usually Keebler crackers with tons of mayo. (You remember Keebler crackers? That giant green cylinder tin flashback.)

When I was around 15, every morning I'd get a bacon, egg, and cheese from the store or from the cart by my school. Always the same: bacon, egg, and cheese on a toasted roll with butter. I also ate a lot of McDonald's back then because they always had a 2 for $3 Big Mac or Quarter Pounder special. I'd usually get a couple items from there for lunch or maybe I'd get pizza. I would buy my loosies (loose cigarettes)—they were only $0.15 each at the time. If you are what you eat, I was just a big ol' pile of garbage.

Let's say you had a completely different experience growing up: Your family had a big-ass garden that you ate fresh fruits and veggies from, or more than once someone said to you, "Here's a plate of green things that grew in the earth—eat them; they're good for you." *You* might eat like shit for different reasons, perhaps because you're rejecting that upbringing or because your friends eat like crap and when you go out you just go with the flow or maybe you create the flow—either way, having a perfectly healthy upbringing doesn't always equal perfectly healthy behaviors when you're on your own.

Consider this moment when you're at brunch with your friends: There you are, you're all eating like crap and looking at each other like *it's all good*, and then you lock eyes with your friend Lola as you're eating your seventh buffalo wing and about to order your fourth mimosa . . . And you sense in this moment that Lola is having the same thought you're having, which is that maybe your group of friends could be better together, you could do something different for a change. *Lola, you reading my mind??* But then it passes, and you make the same plans for next week. Same place? Yeah, bitch, you know I love $5 all-you-can-eat apps.

Listen, so do I. We all love a good deal, especially on foods that tantalize our taste buds at the base level and send out pleasure signals that tell us to eat more (see my favorite childhood eats a few paragraphs ago). But these kinds of good deals offer short-term savings only and will lead to far greater expenses down the road when it comes to your health and how you feel about yourself (usually shitty).

All this stuff—what you learned or didn't learn about food growing up, how you feel you have to eat around certain friends and family because it's just habit or tradition (now, there's a loaded word!)—it's all part of the iceberg of shit. You *use* these things to keep yourself from committing to something that's going to make you better because nothing is better than having a shitload of excuses to feed our insatiable need to self-sabotage. We tell ourselves that we can't help it, "it's just how I was raised . . ." or "it would be rude to order something else . . ." or "I can't bring a salad to the potluck—how boring" or "If I don't get blackout drunk on girls' night, they're gonna think I'm so boring or I actually feel bored . . ." Okay, what's your line? What reason do you use not to do something different that is really just an excuse?

Imma let you think about it for a minute while I talk about one more item in this department.

THE CULT OF COMPARISON

Another thing that I think just about everyone has built into their 'berg is the habit of comparison. So much of how we feel about ourselves today comes by way of comparison.

Disclaimer: I love Instagram. And I use it to share so much, probably too much, about my life. But I never sugarcoat that shit. (I would never sell myself out like that—why steer people the wrong way? I was you! I am you!) My stories show the nitty-gritty, the down and dirty, the . . . camel toe?! No, seriously. I once dedicated a whole story to a "camel toe blocker" that I had to create because people were complaining about having to see my actual real body while I was working out. So basically, people *wish* I would use Photoshop and make my shit look all fake and perfect because that's what they're used to. Crazy. Sorry, kids. My favorite filter is the no-bullshit filter. You're gonna see it all.

Anyyyyway, back to my point, which is to say that comparing yourself to what you see on social media is pointless for two reasons: 1) Those pictures are probably Photoshopped, and definitely posed and filtered, and 2) you will never be anybody but you, so quit trying to be someone else or even spending time wishing you were someone else—the only person you can be is you, but better.

One other reason it's pointless to compare yourself to the 'Gram is the fact that what you don't see matters more than what you do see. What you don't see is the work that everybody, no matter who they are, has to put in to get the body they want. There aren't any kind of Golden Glutes tickets given out at birth (well, except maybe to Arnold Schwarzenegger's kids). Even my girl Kim has to work incredibly hard to get the body she feels good in.

Of course, the question is: Do you have to leave the cult of social media to escape the comparison? I don't think so. Because the truth is that we can easily practice comparison all damn day whether we're online or offline. When you're walking down the street, dogging your neighbor for getting the new car you wanted, or you're in the grocery store glaring at some chick because she has a tight, lifted ass *and* several pints of ice cream in her cart—all you're doing is starin' and comparin'. But just like with social media pics, you don't know the whole story, you just think you do. What you see are only superficial details, and yet that's probably enough to judge the other person, and most definitely yourself. *Why don't I have that car? Why don't I have that ass? Waaaaaaaaah.*

Guess where this kind of thinking gets you? NOWHERETOWN. Every. Single. Time. Is that where you want to live?

Let's face it: There is a cunning sort of appeal to Nowheretown. It's much easier to get wrapped up in what's going on with other people's lives than to deal with our own. We find it irresistible because Nowheretown is smack dab in the middle of the State of Self-Doubt. If we were comfortable in our own skin, felt proud of our own accomplishments and capabilities, the appeal of comparison wouldn't exist.

What's crazy is it seems that almost everyone lives in the State of Self-Doubt—it's a crowded freaking place! Even some of the most beautiful, wealthy, and privileged people reside there, questioning their worthiness and abilities just like the rest of us. I don't know *why* these questions are so common (I'm no Dr. Phil!), but it probably has origins in family or society, or both.

When you reside in the State of Self-Doubt, you don't do any of the things that would make you the best version of yourself. Why? Because it's so much easier to sit back and survey other people's shit, to not take initiative, to not make decisions and be the boss of your life, to follow instead of lead. If you did any of these things, you would lose the opportunity to point your finger at someone or something and you would have to hold yourself responsible. YIKES.

The longer you spend living in this mind-set, the stronger it becomes and the harder it is to leave. But, what you have to realize is that the State of Self-Doubt is mostly self-perpetuated, and it's built by beliefs that aren't true. They only feel true to you because you've allowed them to exist long enough to develop an appearance of truth.

I know for me, when I was growing up, I never had anyone to look up to or someone to say "good job" or "you're so smart . . . talented . . . special." I had none of that, so I filled in those gaps with beliefs that pretty much confirmed the opposite. It wasn't until recently, as part of my own turnaround, that I had to learn how to dig deep and access the super-power we all have called *self-belief*. I had to legit rewire my brain! I had to realize that there is no amount of external validation that could change what or how I thought of myself. Only I could do that; only I could fill my bucket of self-love by doing all those things I thought I couldn't do, all those things I didn't believe I deserved.

It's crazy to think that we keep ourselves in this state of mind because no matter how terrible we feel, it is our comfort zone, it's what we know. The unknown is scary even if it leads to success and happiness.

So, if we can't get away from comparison, what should we do? We start instead to seek out sources of inspiration, comparison's way more positive and productive cousin. If comparison is corroding, inspiration is buffing; it'll bring out the shine in you. People who are inspired are more inclined to begin—and commit to—any kind of journey, whether it is fitness-related or otherwise. People who compare are usually the ones who are looking for the fast way, the hack.

This isn't something I just know intuitively because I'm super deep and shit; it's some-thing I had to learn myself. I definitely fell into both categories in the beginning of my transformation. I compared myself to other girls, or rather to the skinny girls, all the time. I would look at them and think, *I want to be skinny* or *I want to have a flat stomach*. But I had zero clue about what any of these chicks were doing to get their bodies, and I took everything 100% at face value rather than looking deeper into the process. *They must just be doing some sneaky shit that I can't see*, I thought—*I'll just try to take a pill or starve myself and see if that's what they're doing.*

Part of this was probably because I started to compare myself so early on to the five seemingly perfect girls I grew up with. As far as I could tell, none of them were doing any-thing different than me, so there must have been some behind-the-scenes fix that they were all in on.

Of course, I know now that how I responded to all this had a lot to do with a lack of self-confidence. I didn't have a whole lot of love for myself, and a lack of love can leave you more susceptible to comparison. When self-love is missing, it's so much easier to just compare based on quick, surface-level stuff rather than opening your eyes to see the bigger picture.

After years of taking this route (and getting only to Nowheretown), I finally learned that comparison was a dead-end street. So, I started looking for people whose stories showed the deeper work and the deeper truth about what it really takes to achieve great things. I looked for signs of dedication, mental strength, and demonstrations of progress because nothing good comes easy. These were the things that made me feel inspired and made me want to work on myself rather than compare and look for the quick fix.

In the end, it's not about the abs or the chiseled arms or getting the muscular ass, the one you thought you wanted. If you do the work, if you challenge yourself and go through the hardship, sacrifice, and pain and reach each tiny goal every fucking day, you'll realize you don't even care if you have chiseled abs or not. You start to appreciate your body in a whole new way, you start to see YOU and not anyone else, you become your own inspiration—and there's no better feeling than seeing you from the inside out and not the other way around.

What ends up making you happy is never the end result, it's all the stuff in between: It's all the days you woke up early instead of staying in bed and skipping your workout; it's all the cookies you didn't reach for; it's the sweat drops that rolled into your eyes in the 30 minutes you spent on that Stairmaster when you didn't lower the level or get off at 28 minutes. It's all the times you said *yes* to yourself! That right there, my friends, is the goal: self-love. If that is your goal, then happiness is the end result. No waist trainer, no detox, no diet pill will *ever* give you that.

TIME TO MELT THAT ICEBERG

So, you're probably now thinking, *WTF, Mel??! Why you gotta remind me of all the reasons I can't ever get shit done?* I'll tell you why: because now you're going to take all those excuses masquerading as reasons that are all melded together in this below-the-surface megamass that's holding you back and you're going to melt that motherfucker to the ground. There's no way in hell you're going to turn around your life (if you just want to change your body, that's cool, too, but I think you'll be surprised by all the bonus change that comes with) when you've built such a strong case against possibility. You've already lawyered up against yourself!!

I know it sounds kind of meta, this whole iceberg metaphor, but it's just one way for you to think about and visualize all the built-in blame we carry around with us. You can see it as an iceberg, a hard drive—or a pizza covered in toppings where every topping is an excuse . . . *damn you, pepperoni, for making it so hard for me to get my workout in.* Okay, maybe not that—that'll just make you (and me) hungry. Really, though, you can envision it however you like as long as you 1) think about your personal experience and then, 2) mentally collect all the crap you've said to yourself in your head about why you've yet to achieve the body or level of fitness you desire. I'll give you a minute. You could even write all that shit down on paper.

Got it all? Good. Now it's time to forget it all. Melt it down, wipe that hard drive. Imagine it disappearing. If you wrote it on a piece of paper, feel free to burn it. If you feel yourself resisting, I get it. Once you remove all this shit that you've accepted before today because it protected you, you know what's left? A blank page, a raw and vulnerable landscape where it's just you and the brand-new baby promise of opportunity. Holy shit, that's a scary place! I know it. I know what it's like to be confronted face-to-face with yourself and your responsibility for the reality that is your life. You feel alone, you feel scared, but dammit, you are YOU. You are not someone else. And more important, you are not blaming someone or something else anymore for why you're not fit or why you haven't accomplished any other goals in your life.

The unexpected thing that happens when you complete this exercise is that you create room to fall in love with yourself, the real you. *Yeah, that's you.* Let yourself be her, see her. She's fucked up, flawed no doubt, but she ain't got no one else to blame but herself. When you claim her confidently as your own, you will connect for real for maybe the first time and you will create the chance for your life to unfold.

FIT GURL CHAPTER 2 TO-DO LIST

1. **MAKE SURE TO MELT IT.** If you didn't do it already, melt that iceberg of shit to the ground.

2. **START THINKING SUSTAINABILITY.** When I was first starting out on my transformation, I really messed with my head (and my progress) by focusing strictly on weight loss. My thought was *I want to lose (insert weight amount, 10 pounds, 20 pounds, etc.) as FAST as possible!* This is the way most people approach changing their body, but it's not the right way. Start thinking about being healthy and looking hot long term. Whether you're 23, 33, or 53 now, we all have one thing in common: We are all getting older! And shit gets hard as you get older. So think about creating habits that will benefit you for years and years, no matter what your starting point is.

3. **LEARN TO USE A NEW SCALE.** If you have a certain number you want to see on the scale, you must remember:

   • The number doesn't move if you don't.

   • The number means nothing if you feel good.

   • If you don't know what you want, start with what you know you don't want.

   • Losing weight requires eating.

   • You're more than just a number on a scale!

4. **MIND MUSCLES MATTER, TOO.** Another early mistake I made was separating the physical strength from the mental strength; I was working on both simultaneously and not even realizing it. I really think paying attention to your mental space and working on your mental strength is so important (as you can probably tell from these first two chapters). In fact, I think this stuff is just as essential to The Turnaround as the workouts.

Chapter Three

The Four C's That Will Set You Free

Control, Connection, Concentration, and Consistency

Straight talk: This book is here to help you achieve a rocking physical transformation, which is no doubt your goal in reading this. You want to see your hottest, strongest, sexiest self staring back at you in the mirror; you want to walk by a store window and catch the reflection of your ass and think, *Damn, that's ME!* I get that that's your goal, and your ass will be in the gym working on creating that reflection before you know it—and then you'll only be wishing you were back here reading these cute little words on the page instead of standing in a room full of sweaty people holding a giant hunk of metal in your hand and busting out rep after rep after rep. Trust me on this.

But for right now, we're going to keep working on your mental prep. People don't talk enough about the fact that getting to the physical transformation you want takes so much more than just doing specific exercises or following the right combination of sets and reps; it requires an awareness of all kinds of invisible influences that have a major impact on your success (or lack of it).

In this last chapter before we get to the program, I want to bring some of these influences out into the open by introducing you to the Four C's, a collection of what I've found to be the most important behavioral elements of success: Control, Connection, Concentration, and Consistency. Each of these will play a role in helping you create intentional habits that are good for you—which, let's be honest, seem to be way harder to create than those that are bad for us.

If you're like I was when I first started, you're in a space where you're almost addicted to feeling bad, or you've at least become accustomed to the discomfort and are so set on the direction you're headed in that you can't see things being any other way. STOP! You're not stuck, you have a CHOICE (another C-word that's vital and extremely important for you to be aware of). You don't think you have a choice? Well, I'm sorry to break it to you, but choosing and *not* choosing are choices. So the next time you don't take control and you put your life into something or someone else's hands, that was all YOU. Think about that.

I want you to imagine all the things you can do with choice. You can tell your boss to fuck off—maybe not out loud or exactly like that, but you can say, "No, I'm not staying late today." You can *not* smoke that cigarette. And that french fry you're holding up to your mouth? You can put that fry down because it doesn't have arms or legs or a persuasive tongue stronger than your own.

It's not easy, but everything you do—from where you sleep, to what time you wake up, to the type of toothbrush you use, to where you park your car, to every step you take and where those steps lead to—are *choices*. No matter what your circumstances, I want you to know that YOU HAVE A CHOICE, and you are the driver of your life. If you don't like the road you're on, keep driving down that road and complaining as you go, but if you're ready to see something different, then get off at the next exit, because you aren't anywhere close to your final destination.

It's time to wake up and smell the C's.

1. CONTROL

Transformation begins with realizing you have control of your life. This may sound like the most obvious statement ever, but most people don't truly know they have control over their own actions—because if they did, they wouldn't constantly be saying that they can't make time to exercise, can't eat healthy, can't do whatever it is they actually want to do. Oh, really? You don't say. Well, that's funny because somehow you found a way to say, "I can sit in front of the TV for three hours every night" or "I can eat 3,000 calories of creamy fettucine alfredo for dinner and top it off with a bottle of wine and some cannolis for dessert." You CANed all over that shit. But making time for a workout? Nope. There's no way in hell I can do that.

Think about it. We are faced with hundreds of small decisions and questions every day and, whether you realize it or not, you have control each time to decide what you want to do. And, each time, you have the option to choose the action or to make the decision that will benefit you the most. What we do *is* completely up to us, but we usually don't take the time to consider this because we are so stuck in our default operating mode.

And this default mode is crazy stubborn and usually supported by the incorrect beliefs that we're in too deep or we're too late to make a change. But every moment presents another opportunity to do the right thing for yourself. Even if you can't see it yet, there is always a right option in every decision you make.

You can start to break out of your default mode by consciously taking the time to ask yourself something that you know the answer to deep down: What is really going to make me the best version of myself or the ME I want to be, the person I already am inside, the one who isn't hiding behind the fog? You might have expected this question to be more along the lines of "What's going to make me happy?" but you're not ready for that—you don't know what that means just yet. I say this because I remember a time in my own life when I would have said that smoking my cigarettes and having my sugar-filled coffee made me "happy," but the deeper reality was that I only felt worse about myself every day. Don't settle for the superficial, quick-fix answer. Go deeper to where the real truth hides. You know the true answer.

After you have your answer, I want you to at least once make the choice to do the thing that is going to put you on the path to that best version. I'll hold your spot on this page while you go do that thing . . .

Didn't that feel good? Now do it again. See this as the beginning of a new pattern that you can replicate. You don't have to be perfect at it right away; you have to learn to make the choice that will make your life better. It all starts with just one better choice. For me, it was skipping the cigarette with sugar coffee and instead making breakfast at home and drinking some water. Those were baby, baby steps, but I could feel I was at the beginning of something new.

Speaking of smoking, it definitely taught me about the power of choice the hard way. I smoked for a long time. I also wanted to quit for a long time, and I always felt like I was trying to quit. I would quit for one day and it would feel so good, but there was always a trigger that I would accept as a reason I could start again: *Something shitty happened, I can smoke again*, I'd think in my head. It was a constant battle. I always had a rock-solid justification for why I could break my promise to myself and smoke one more. I must have told myself a thousand times: "I'm having a bad day; I'll smoke a few cigarettes and get back to my stuff tomorrow, fresh."

A lot of people go through this same cycle with exercise, except *not* exercising is their bad habit. Instead of saying, "I'll stop smoking when I feel better," you might say, "I'll start exercising when I feel better." The problem is, no one feels better until they take the action that is going to equal feeling better.

Even if you're not addicted to nicotine, you're probably addicted to the voice of "Not-Today Nancy." Oh, you don't know Not-Today Nancy? She's that little voice in your head that says don't work out today, don't eat healthy today, don't start your business or meditate or drink water or do yoga today. She'll also say things like, "Remember that thing that happened earlier that made you kinda sad/tired/yucky? You deserve to eat a pint of ice cream!" Not-Today Nancy is a little like a two-faced "friend" who says nice things to your face, but behind your back is really trying to destroy you. Except Nancy is doing all her dirty work from the inside. It's time to kick this B out of your head: *Hey, Nancy! Your lease is up, and I'm not renewing!*

What's strange is that it would seem that doing what's good for you would be the easiest thing in the world. Yet, most of us are so fucked up that we are almost addicted to feeling bad—and I don't mean that as a criticism of you as an individual. It's almost like it's part of the human condition to feel comfortable in discomfort. It's the same as when people stay in shitty relationships or crap jobs forever because it's just what they know.

The million-dollar question is how do you break out of the comfort zone, aka your default mode? You grab the wild, powerful dragon called *control* by its horns and you ride that thing like you're motherfuckin' Khaleesi.

Or, back in real life, you start by admitting that you have all the control. This isn't a small thing, mostly because control has a conjoined twin called *responsibility*; when you admit that you're in control you also have to take full responsibility for your actions. And I don't mean that you've got to be responsible like having to pay your bills and shit like that.

I mean that it's time to acknowledge that you are a full-on adult who is responsible for 1) the living, breathing being that is you, and 2) the big and small decisions you make each day that add up to creating this you.

Accepting responsibility requires a radical brand of honesty with yourself that might feel a little bit uncomfortable at first. There's no room for lies. Do you know what's going to happen when you stick to your current habits of excuse-making, justification, self-punishment? You bet your ass you know what's going to happen. The same damn shit, day after day.

These aren't just empty thoughts or mental exercises without purpose—we have a goal here, people! And that goal is to begin to build trust in yourself to do what's in your own best interest. *Build* is the key word here—you've got to work a little to become your own BFF again. Think of it like you're reconnecting with a friend who treated you like shit before, but she's saying she's changed, and you're saying, "Okay, I'm going to give you another chance, but we're going to take it slow. I want to see proof that you're for real going to look out for me." (You might not think you've treated yourself like shit, but if you haven't been taking care of your body, you definitely haven't been doing yourself any favors.)

So, how do you prove to yourself that you're really taking the reins this time, that you're in control and taking responsibility for your destiny? You start by creating a humble new habit that's just for you. Something that you choose to do differently and that is part of the new version of you that you want to create.

Here's what I started doing *for me* every morning: waking up at 4:00 a.m. to make my coffee. I know it might sound crazy to wake up that early, but doing so has proved to be a gift I give to myself each day. I get up and boil water for my Chemex, which is this cool hourglass-shaped glass carafe that's used for making coffee. The filter and coffee grinds chill right at the opening at the top. When the water's the right temperature, I pour it over the waiting coffee grinds in slow, meditative circles. It's the best! As I do this, I feel a calmness come over me no matter what's going on in my life.

The coffee takes 20 minutes to brew, and I feel like a kid on Christmas morning every single day waiting for it to be done. What I've found, though, is that this is an awesome way to help build patience and concentration. I swear, the more you think about your coffee, the better it's going to be—concentrating on its goodness will enrich it. By the time it's done, that coffee will taste like the best damn thing you've ever had in your life.

My pre-day-getting-started time wasn't always as calm as it is now, especially when I first started working out. I initially tried fitting my workouts in during the mornings, but this just made for total chaos. So then I tried making time for workouts after work. It never stuck. I came to the realization that to make it work I had to just get up at 5:00 a.m. I could just get my ass up and do what I fucking needed to do. And I did it, and that's pretty much been my schedule ever since.

Of course, now I'm fortunate in that a lot of mornings I get to train others, but I think transitioning into doing that as my job would have felt way rougher if I didn't already have the same sort of pattern in my day. Even when it feels rough to get up super early—and trust me, there are mornings when it does—I just tell myself that in 10 minutes I'm going to feel better.

Before you start creating your workout schedule, I want you to establish a little habit for yourself. Create a "brewing" ritual of your own, except it doesn't have to actually be making coffee—just something that you can commit to each day that demonstrates you have control of your life. You could meditate or journal or read, or dedicate 30 minutes to starting your own business, working on a side hustle. Find and perfect your little craft. It will become just what you need.

Once you've started creating your habit of choice, try to reflect on it and see how it affects your day.

Other Ways to Start Taking Control

- **ASK YOURSELF: DO ALL MY MICRO-DECISIONS MATCH UP WITH MY BIG DREAMS?** Just about every decision you make has a cumulative effect. Are your decisions contributing to the creation of the life you want? Remember: no more lies.

- **STOP WAITING FOR THE YELLOW BRICK ROAD TO THE LIFE OF YOUR DREAMS.** You've gotta build that shit yourself. Ticktock. I don't care if you're 23 or 63. It's time to get to work.

- **DON'T TRY TO MAKE TIME—IT'S NOT SOMETHING YOU CAN JUST COOK UP IN THE KITCHEN—TAKE TIME FOR YOURSELF.** You have to take time, otherwise someone or some excuse will take it for you. Don't allow anyone or anything to get in your way.

- **BE PREPARED TO BREAK THE RULES BY BEING EXACTLY WHO YOU WANT TO BE!** You are in control, which means:

- If you want to lift weights, do it.

- If you want to fight MMA, do it.

- If you want to be a lumberjack, do it! (Damn, I wanna be a lumberjack.)

- If you want to take up quilting *and* rock some killer quads at the same damn time, DO IT.

You are strong.
You are smart.
You are beautiful.
You can do anything you want.
You are in control.

Don't ever let anyone put you down or tell you otherwise. If they don't like you for who you are or who you want to be, throw on your fuck-'em shoes and walk out the damn door. Because life is short and ain't nobody got time for that!

2. CONNECTION

In a lot of ways, The Turnaround is about creating a new relationship with yourself. And you cannot have a strong relationship with yourself without connection.

To forge a renewed connection, you first have to get to know your body, this thing you spend all your time in. So many people I meet want to know how I did it, how I changed my body, and I tell them, "I had to wake up and be honest with myself—I was disconnected." I didn't know anything about my body; I didn't know how to care for it; I didn't know or care to know anything about the food I was eating. And I let myself stay stuck in that confusion for so long because I didn't want to learn. I didn't want to pay attention.

But you can't transform your body or your life from that space. I had to get to know myself in a deeper way if I wanted to evolve, and that required clearing out the mental clutter made up of expectations and negative self-talk, and the physical mess created by all the crap foods I was eating. Only then was I able to connect to my true potential and start to bring it to life.

I believe the same is true for you. Not to say you're going to clean up your shit and get connected and suddenly become a hard-core fitness junkie like me, a crazy lady who lives in workout clothes and gets to call the gym her office—that was *my path*.

What's your path? Maybe it's still to be discovered, or maybe you're on it and it's just so overgrown with weeds you can no longer see which way to go. Regardless, working on your own turnaround will help you start to see the path to your potential light up like the Vegas Strip.

It might seem like a reach to say that starting a workout program will lead you to some greater sense of direction or purpose, but I've seen it happen, and not just in my own life. When you dedicate time to taking care of yourself, it's like forced bonding time. Even if you work out with a buddy or a trainer, you are on your own with those weights. You have to push, pull, lug, and lift that shit all by yourself. You get to know your body in an intimate way, and you start to trust and really like yourself because you begin to see capability and courage; you feel energized and empowered. And *these* are the lights that help you start to see your potential in other areas of your life.

What's really interesting is that when you're doing the work, the space in your head for distractions such as unrealistic expectations and superficial destinations (e.g., "I just want

Body by Mel

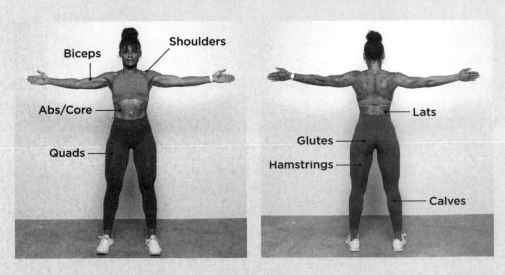

to get to six-pack abs!") gets smaller and smaller. That's because the thoughts of appreciation for what you're accomplishing in the moment and the day-to-day progress you're making start to move in and take up space.

Now, just like any new relationship, this one is going to get a little physical—not *sexual*, just physical. So, I want you to touch yourself. (I said not like that. Sheesh.) Just touch your body: your shoulders, your biceps, your forearms, your belly, your butt, quads, calves. Get to know it. Even those parts that have always bothered you, the ones you've always told your BF or GF to stay away from ("Ugh, I told you I don't like your hands on my stomach . . ."). Feel your body. Without judgment. Feel your hip joints, knees, elbows—you know, all those awesome bendy things that make so much of your movement possible. You might even journal about this process and what comes up for you when you do it.

Here's why I want you to do this—nothing strengthens connection more than physical touch; that's just how human beings work. Plus, when you create this tangible sort of familiarity with all your parts, it will accelerate your ability to boss your body around once you start hitting the gym. Maybe if you're lucky, yours will start taking your call sooner than mine did!

Other Ways to Create and Improve Connection

- **USE KNOWLEDGE TO BUILD A BETTER BOND WITH YOUR BODY.** Don't be shy about studying the body glossary you just saw. This will help you understand which body parts you're using in each exercise. Besides, when someone says, "nice hammies," you'll want to know what the heck they're talking about.

- **START THINKING ABOUT THE FOODS YOU EAT EVERY DAY.** It's not time yet for you to make any changes to your diet, so don't stress . . . But do start paying attention to what you eat each day. And ask yourself these questions:

  - How much of what I eat is fresh food that was grown in the dirt or in a tree?

  - How much of what I eat comes from a box or a plastic bag that I could pop? (Anything with air means it's processed!)

    If you are eating a lot of stuff with chemicals, that is, any and all processed foods, you're going to have to get real with your foods when the time comes. Not just yet—but get ready.

- **TAKE A GROUP WORKOUT CLASS.** It might sound counterintuitive to suggest this, but putting yourself into the middle of a workout class can enhance self-connection. This is because you're going to feel a little self-conscious, which is something we've been taught to think of as a bad thing, but I want you to use it to your advantage. I want you to take that awkwardness or fear you feel around doing stuff you're not super familiar with in front of other people and turn it into an intense form of focus on your efforts. (Pretend you're in *X-Men* or *Supergirl* or some other show like that). If you work on connecting with yourself in this setting, you will emerge with some serious self-confident swag. You might also create some connections with other people who, like you, are also working on themselves and may end up supporting and encouraging your success—how cool would that be?! A big part of this journey is inward, but that doesn't mean you always have to be alone while you're on it.

3. CONCENTRATION

So, concentration is kind of a big deal these days—and by big deal, I mean it's super fucking hard to concentrate in today's world. Mostly because we have these tiny little computers called smartphones pretty much surgically implanted in our hands that we stare at all day. And when we're not staring at them, we're thinking about staring at them (my phone is across the table from me as I'm trying to write and we're having a legit staring contest). We are definitely addicted—to where these phones take us; to ventures into other people's lives and the clothes they wear, the places they go; to information we *need to know immediately* (what time does Shake Shack open?).

The specifics of your information intake don't matter because whatever it is, it's in addition to all the other crap in your actual life—all your own work and family stuff, schedule challenges, car trouble, pet problems, the constant questions: *What do you want for dinner? Did you do laundry? Did you get those new pants for that interview next week? Did you send your sister a birthday card? What TV show do you wanna watch? AAaaaackrrrrrghhhhh.*

The point is, we all have a fuckton of shit swimming in and out of our heads every minute of every day. And fighting through all that mess to concentrate on any one thing feels damn near impossible. But let me tell you something that I've discovered: Working out offers one of the few tickets to freedom from all the noise because it demands not just your presence, but your focus, too. Especially working out with weights, where concentration and respect are required if you really want to get something out of it (and if you don't want to get hurt!).

People often make the mistake of thinking that working out with weights means just moving them in a repetitive pattern. But I always tell my clients, "If that's what you think, then you have already lost 70% of your investment in getting fit." There is so much more to it, and so many teeny-tiny details to concentrate on, which equals so many opportunities to create progress and change in your body.

When performing exercises, the most important thing is to be aware of your body and how it moves. During a squat, for example: the position of your feet (make sure you're firmly grounded), how your knees are flexing (they shouldn't wobble left and right), how low you're coming down with your hips (thighs at least parallel with the floor), where your shoulders, elbows, chest, and head are pointing . . . These *all* affect the quality of every single rep. See what I mean? Lots of opportunity to check out from all that other crap in your life and check in on yourself. For about an hour or so—can you give yourself that time?

There can be extreme and long-lasting consequences to not paying attention to or concentrating on these details. That may sound dramatic, but it's the absolute truth— when you are distracted or detached from the details of your workout, you're not going to get the results you want. This will lead first to feeling bummed, second to giving up, and worst of all, thinking that you've tried and failed, when really you just haven't tried the right way. This sets up a convincing narrative of self-doubt that can make you shut the door on second chances, potentially shaping the rest of your life as it relates to your health and fitness. That's not your story. Nope.

To ensure that's not your story, you've got to start the workouts ready to concentrate on what you're doing. In the beginning, it might feel challenging, especially when you're trying to learn all the details of the exercises, but just attach yourself like a barnacle to those details—don't give in to the part of you that senses the demand on your attention and tries to tempt you into distractions. Stay on task. I swear, it's almost like you have to retrain your brain, but you can do it and when you do, you will be rewarded beyond measure.

You'll start to experience these rewards even after the first workout, when you have this moment of feeling so fully in the present, so free from all those other thoughts, that it'll hit you like the fourth sip of a brunch cocktail—yep, it'll be a little bit buzzy. Sure, your muscles might be burning at the same time (unlike when you're at brunch), but you'll see—it's a special sort of salvation, one that you will grow to savor.

How to Concentrate

- **STOP (LITERALLY) PHONING IN YOUR REPS.** I don't mean to harp on the phone thing, but seriously—don't do four shitty reps and then check your texts or IG! Commit, get off your phone, and move with intention and focus. Every single second of intensity and focus you put into your training will yield far greater results than a bunch of random moves practiced without full concentration. If you feel like you've gotta check IG or whatever, use the 45 seconds between sets to do so. Although, I will say that if you don't need those 45 seconds to shake out your muscles and catch your breath, you may want to check yourself and make sure you're working hard enough.

- **SLOW DOWN.** If you still feel like you're having trouble concentrating on your workouts, try slowing down. It's a simple strategy, but probably the best approach to improving your exercise quality. Take it slow and think about how each muscle is moving and bring deep awareness to your breath. Even if this means carving out a little more time for your workouts initially, it will be worth it. (And it won't be forever—you'll get into a groove.)

- **USE YOUR CALENDAR.** In order to free up space in your brain for concentrating on the things that matter, you've got to value time, and the best way to put a value on time is to save it. Think about it. You might save a special weekend that you want to have with your dude or lady or with your family, but we usually don't think about saving time for ourselves—and we're almost ashamed to say so, even if we do. When was the last time you heard someone say, "No, sorry, I'm going to leave that time open for a date with myself"? I would say, "Hell, yeah!" to that. But usually we have to make up some shit like a doctor's appointment to excuse our self-care time.

  I suggest doing more time saving in general. Set aside time—actually block it out in your calendar for your workouts, for a recovery massage, for a facial, for a fucking lunch by yourself if that would make you happy, and for all the things that matter most to you in your life. If you haven't called your family/parents/siblings in a while or spent some time alone with your best friend, save the time now for those things. You won't regret it. Plus, you'll find that once you've set aside the time, you'll be more present and able to concentrate on the moment when it arrives because you've given yourself permission in advance to have it.

- **EYES ON YOUR OWN PLATE.** Don't concentrate *all* your efforts on gym time; what's on your plate matters just as much! Be present with your food—so many people scarf down snacks and meals without even realizing what they've eaten. Try having one meal without your TV on and without your phone in your hand. Engage in conversation or just enjoy your meal. We are so programmed to make meals into multitasking events, whereas the act of eating a meal is in and of itself an event.

4. CONSISTENCY

So, this final C isn't exactly a topic that will get a girl pumped up. By definition, consistency is about predictability, routine, and simply showing up again and again and again. Kind of a *yawn*. Yet consistency is perhaps the most important factor in creating a legitimate and lasting life turnaround. Being consistent with your workouts is a profound act of self-love.

A lot of us think consistently carving out this time just for us feels selfish, but what my fitness journey taught me was that to be there for my family and others, I had to be there for myself first. I had to love myself first.

I think in our heads we can't always get the math of this—the logical thing is to think that the more time dedicated to other people, the better; it shows them how much we care. But this constant state of energy going outward is a drain. You have to restore and recharge. Getting time to do this on the calendar is great, as I suggested, but it's more than that—it's a mind-set, too. You've got to start thinking that putting "me first" is allowed.

This is a mind-set that those around you have to start adopting as well, but you've got to lead the change. You have to teach people that you are someone who is committed to your own self-care, and believe it or not, they will learn to see you that way. They will learn to respect your commitment, your consistency, and you won't have to work at it anymore. Trust me. They'll start saying things like, "Oh right, you gotta get your workout in . . . I'll grab the kid/the groceries/etc." (This might not happen until after you've had to yell a dozen times, but it WILL happen—as long as you are consistent in your commitment.)

One of the things I noticed as I became more dedicated to achieving my goals was that I was naturally more mindful of other people, too. I started to value my time so much that I wanted to make sure that I fully valued that of others. I wasn't a big jerk before I started making good on commitments to myself (okay, maybe sometimes, if I'm being totally honest), but I do feel that having a little more self-awareness helped me have more general awareness, too.

Since I want things done with quality, I started to make sure quality was the driver of the work that I put out, whether it's a training program or giving an interview. I've also become more patient with the world after learning that I need to be patient with myself and my results. More important, literally every day, I learn the value of having positive, loving thoughts, since that affects our perception of what happens in our lives. Having this mind-set helps you see the opportunities for improvement rather than the setbacks.

Now, I know I'm throwing out a lot of buzzwords here like *self-awareness, self-care, commitment, consistency,* but this shit is all meaningless if it's just left here on the page. Seriously, all this stuff is just going to sit here in this same damn spot on the same damn page for eternity. The only way it will ever have any value is if you start acting it out in your real life. If you were reading the script of your life, it would be time for you to read the line that says, "I must do good shit for myself every day." So Shakespearean, I know. Say it out loud wherever you are. I dare you.

The hard truth is that being consistent with a habit, even one you grow to love, is tough work. I don't want to sugarcoat it because you've already heard plenty of lies, or fibs, about it before: "It's super easy! Just put a sticky on your mirror and you'll make your dreams happen." No. Sorry, it doesn't work like that. You have to fight for consistency, fight as hard as you would for a really fucking amazing relationship. You have to care for, value, and love yourself just as much as you would another person—even more, because this is the only relationship that will last you your entire life. You are the only one you can say 100% you'll have forever. So, be good to you.

How to Create Consistency

- **BE RELIABLE AND DEPENDABLE—TO YOURSELF.** We are so much more inclined to drop the ball on promises we make to ourselves than on those we make to others. It's time to start sticking to your commitments to *you.*

- **SET GOALS.** I didn't grow up playing sports and never really considered myself an athlete, but when I started working out, I looked to athletes for mind-set guidance. Athletes establish goals, consistently show up to train, and accept failure as part of success. You don't have to be an athlete to benefit from this formula! Just put it into practice.

- **JUST SHOW THE FUCK UP.** Want to stay motivated? Be consistent! There's nothing more motivating than feeling and watching the well-earned results of your dedication. I promise you that motivation will be 1,000% stronger when you are consistent about showing up.

- **CREATE SIMPLE HABITS THAT LEAD TO CONSISTENCY.** Wake up and get up! Yes, just jump out of bed when you hear the alarm. Take that "brewing" habit you created in the first C—Control—and DO THE SAME RITUAL first thing every morning. I make my coffee every day. What little gift are you going to give to yourself every day?

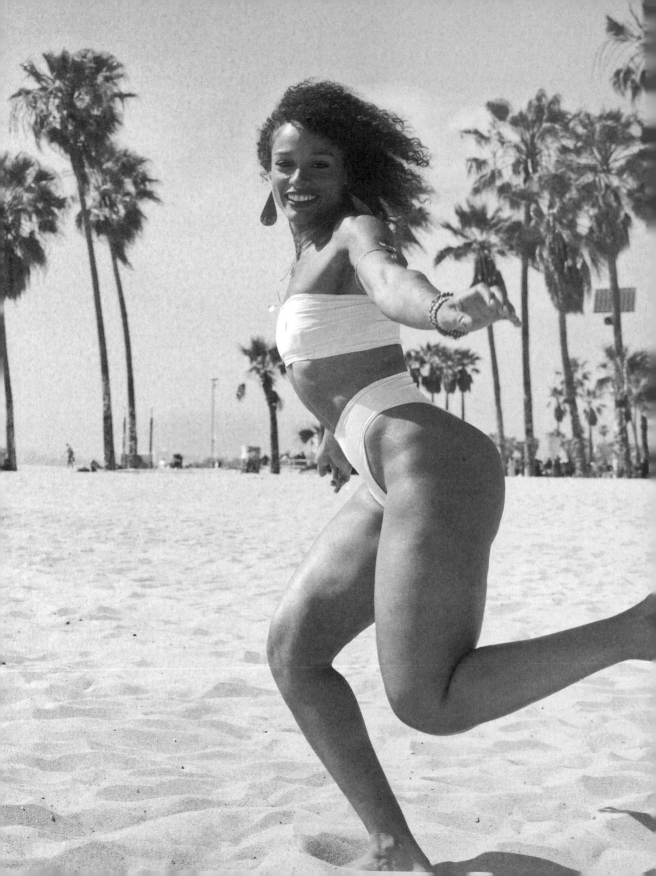

Part Two
The Turnaround

So here we are, boys and girls (mostly girls, amirite?): You've arrived at the program. This is where the magic happens. Well, that's not true—it doesn't literally happen right here on this page. In fact, nothing happens here. Everything I'm writing is worth exactly zero times zero infinity squared (or $(0*0\infty)2=0$ for those of you who are into math) without *you* and your energy, without your beautiful and ugly efforts, your trials and try-agains, your grit and hard-ass work—all of which when dedicated to this program will bring it to life. And that's where the magic happens. In your life, where you take those sleepy dreams of yours and you WAKE THEM THE FUCK UP. It's magic, but it's no miracle: There ain't no pills or prayer that'll take the place of work, so get ready.

Here's how it will work over the next three chapters: You've got three rotations to complete: 45°, 90°, and 180°. Once you've finished these, you've finished turning your shit around. The complete program is 24 working weeks with two non-working (i.e., free) weeks mixed in for recovery, bringing it to a grand total of 26 weeks. That might seem like a long time to you, and guess what? It is a long time. But it's not as long as a life spent lugging around unfulfilled potential will feel.

What will help you not just do it, but do it right, is reading everything I'm including in the rotation chapters, all the nooks and crannies, the nitty-gritty. Each chapter will include some opening info about important food stuff (Mouth), your mental space (Mind), and a little workout commentary (Muscle). This info is like the boots-on-the-ground intel that will help you before you go to battle. All of it was pulled from my personal experience as I made progress (including pep talks I wish someone had given me!) or from input I've received from clients I've trained, whether in person or through workout plans and apps. Don't skip these goodies.

After these setup sections, you'll get into the weekly calendars, in which I'll share the actionable stuff with you: mind-set practices; meal prep, planning, and sample days; and the actual workouts. The workouts will appear written out just the way a trainer would give them to you, and the exercise database beginning on page 197 will serve as your reference guide for how to do each exercise. It may seem tedious at first to look at the descriptions and pictures for exercise instruction, but think of it like you're learning a new language—at first, you might need to use your handbook regularly for help, but then as you gain familiarity with terms and names, you'll kind of just start knowing what to do. You'll know what plyo (plyometric) split lunges, Bulgarian split squats, and sumo dead lifts with one-second holds are; you'll know exactly how to do them all, along with dozens of other exercises; and you'll be able to execute them on command.

WHAT YOU NEED TO GET STARTED

Before you get started, I want to share with you what I call The Turnaround Recipe for Success, aka the long-ass list of shit you *don't* need to get going with your workouts and the short list of what you *truly* need to get your sweat on.

The Turnaround Recipe for Success

No protein powder

No creatine

No branched-chain amino acids (BCAAs)

No fat burners

No fucking waist trainers

Or detox tea

Or detox anything

No drugs

No BULLSHIT!

Your life doesn't need to get all crazy complicated with this BS. You don't *need* anything but this right here:

Time	Intensity
Consistency	Commitment
Dedication	Fucking PATIENCE

And, of course . . . real fucking food—not protein bars and shakes and juicing and dumb shit of that nature.

Oh, and you need one more thing: a goal.

So many of us start a project or program with a "goal" as clear as dirty bathwater, but we don't follow through because we can't even see our own toes, let alone where we're going! (Gross I know, but I bet you really get what I'm sayin' . . .)

An undefined goal equals no real intention or investment. But that's not how it's going to work with The Turnaround. You are going to do the things that are necessary to show up and complete this program to the best of your ability. And one of those things is stopping right here and now and deciding on and defining your goal. It doesn't have to be crazy, but it must rest somewhere on the border between realistic and ambitious. Your goal should also be specific enough so that you can measure against it later on.

Here's an example of a half-ass goal (not good enough) and one that's specific enough to pass The Turnaround test (good enough):

HALF-ASS GOAL: I want to lose some weight in the next six months.

REALISTIC-AMBITIOUS GOAL: I want to follow Mel's training program and food guidelines for at least a 90% adherence for the next six months and lose 25 pounds of unneeded fat, while making some good-looking-ass muscles and finally being able to do a pull-up.

Why do I ask you to find the realistic-ambitious border for your goal? If your story is similar to mine, then you're at a place where you may honestly think you know what you want, but what you want is actually based on what you've been conditioned to think you want.

For example, when I embarked on this pursuit, I wanted to be 125 pounds and I had an image in my head of what I'd look like and how I'd feel walking around at 125 pounds. And I'd see myself eventually accomplishing this goal, and thinking, *Yay, I'm fulfilled AF now and just going to turn on cruise control, right?* NOT HOW IT HAPPENED AT ALL. Once at this goal and while trying to maintain it, I realized that at 125 pounds my body doesn't feel very good, and that I need to manipulate my food to unhealthy levels in order to sustain that. I felt weak and unhealthy—because I was—and the image I had in my head versus reality was so far apart. Turns out that my body feels the best around 135 to 140 pounds. That's when I'm strong, feel clear, and my relationship with food is as healthy as my muscles.

I'm not saying this will be exactly your experience, but I want you to be open to something similar or something surprising happening. Meaning, be ready to learn a ton about yourself and your body.

I've made every effort to ensure that your training and food approach is as sustainable as possible so that it can help you equalize goals that may or may not be where your body wants to be and your mind feels happy. So, don't stress. Write down your goal, babe!

A Note on How to Use the Calendars

In the three rotation chapters, you'll discover a calendar for each week of the program. In most cases, these calendars will provide a week's worth of coaching—this is true except for the weeks where you will be repeating a previous week's workout; these will be shorter. The coaching for each week will look like this:

- The calendar will always open with a MOUTH note—I recommend you read this because if there are any nutrition changes to be made over the upcoming week, that's where you'll find out about it.

- Next, you'll see a MIND note that will speak to where your head may be at during that particular week—or I might just shout out some support, so you know I'm cheering you on all day, every day.

- Then, the workouts will appear under MUSCLE, and these will be progressive. As your performance and skills develop so will your work and recovery load—you'll start with four training sessions per week, then five, then five plus one rest-and-recovery day by the time you're moving like a gazelle and lifting like a gorilla.

Try to keep the workout days connected in the way they're presented—that is, don't insert rest days in between workout days. That said, if you *must* miss a workout, don't panic, but be sure to get it done within the same seven-day period.

Chapter Four

45°

MIND

I've already thrown a lot of information your way, and now I'm about to drop a shit-ton more. But before I do, I just want to say that I know what it's like to be on the receiving end of this much info, and to feel confused as fuck about what to do with all of it. When I was at the beginning, I definitely had no idea where it was going to lead me, or if it was going to go anywhere at all. Which is why I want to tell you two things real quick:

1. Trust me when I say everything is going to fall into place. I know how tough that is to believe at this moment, but just try it—what have you got to lose?? Take the information I'm giving you and bring it to life through your efforts and see what happens. Take a chance on change.

2. You don't have to study all this info and memorize it like you're about to go white-knuckle it through the SAT or GRE or LSAT or some other stressful shit like that. Even just absorbing a little of it is enough; putting it into practice matters most of all, and nothing you do has to be done perfectly in order for you to create progress.

I'm going to suggest that you do something that you may not be the biggest fan of. I want you to take a "before" picture. I know some people are going to hate me for making them do this, but it has to happen. A concrete visual starting point will allow you to see your

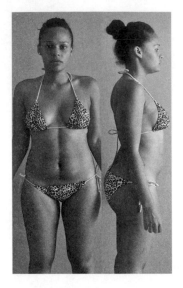

progress objectively. (We are so hard on ourselves that if we try to rely on our own reflection in the mirror as a "progress report," we may never see the amazing changes taking place.)

I want you to make a mental note of how it makes you feel to take these images and to look at them. I know you may see yourself in images all day long thanks to social media, but in a way the pictures we share on social media are for other people—their *reactions* are for us, but we post first for others. The pictures I want you to take and your reaction to them are for you alone. Not in a shameful, secretive way, but in a sacred, seizing-control-of-your-own-story sort of way. Take them and take them in, then use your response to get to know yourself a little better.

You might also consider literally making note of this experience and what it brings up for you. Put your thoughts down in a journal or in the Notes section of your phone, or send an email to yourself. You could also use this as an opportunity to add your "on-the-surface" goals—for example, "tight and toned thighs," "visible abs," etc.

Again, goals of this type really only work like the dangling carrot to get the donkey started, but as you work through the program what you want to achieve will change and evolve more than you can ever imagine. The surface-level goals will end up feeling secondary to the sort of bigger-picture rewards: the changes you'll notice in how you feel about yourself, your confidence, and your bulked-up inner strength. Right now, you think you know the change you want—but you'll see. There's so much more out there.

MOUTH

So, I haven't talked a lot about food yet and there's a reason for it—it can be such a loaded topic, especially for the ladies. And listen, I'm not singling out women in some lazy-ass generalization; I'm speaking from experience in dealing with myself and so many other women over the years: Food can fuck with us more than just about anything else.

In Chapter 1, I shared what I ate growing up and the terrible food habits I carried into my early twenties, but I haven't mentioned my time with what was likely an undiagnosed eating disorder. (I'm 100% certain we're not meant to survive off just processed food and cigarettes, as I did for years.) I don't want to go down this rabbit hole too far because I want to get to how you will want to eat while following this program, but I do have a few important general tips I want to make about food and The Turnaround:

1. **IF YOU LOVE FOOD, FOR THE LOVE OF GOD, KEEP LOVING FOOD.** There's no shame in loving to eat, and truthfully you will not succeed on this program unless you eat enough food. Sure, you may need to swap out some of your staples—but those muscles and tissues you'll be working so hard will need to be fed. And I'm not talking about just SlimFast shakes and other types of synthetic foods; I'm talking about the real deal: rice, chicken, sweet potatoes, veggies, beans, broccoli, cashews—you know, real foods, stuff that comes from trees and dirt.

2. **GET TO KNOW THOSE REAL FOODS, REAL QUICK.** I've found that the fastest way to familiarize yourself with real foods and feel good about what you're eating is to start to prep and cook foods for yourself. This gives you more of a full sensory experience—touch the foods you prep, smell them, taste them raw (unless it's meat!), then taste them cooked. Make eating for the results you want about more than just putting nutrients in your mouth and swallowing them. By the way, digestion starts in the mouth, and the salivation and chewing process is essential to this. So, if you thought you could just drink your nutrients, think again!

3. **THE FOODS YOU EAT ARE THE RAW MATERIALS FOR YOUR FUTURE BODY (NOT TO MENTION BRAIN).** We're all smart enough to know that the whole "you are what you eat" thing is not literal (if it was, my fingers would be fucking french fries by now). But there is a serious truth in this overused phrase, and that is the fact that the quality of what you put in your body matters—a LOT.

4. **THERE'S NO RULE THAT SAYS YOU HAVE TO TAKE YOUR DIET BAGGAGE WITH YOU.** Who cares what you've tried before or what you've failed at or what diet your friend swears by—seriously, let all that shit go. There are so many other areas of life, like love and relationships and family, that are so stuffed full of uncontrollable, unpredictable stress and complications that it just makes no sense at all to let what you eat be another one of them. I'll do my part to try to make it as easy as possible for you to eat in a way that will help you get the best results, but it's up to you to let a little air out of the subject.

Now that I've covered some general food mind-set stuff, let's get into the specifics of the diet strategy I suggest you use while following this program. One feature of my approach is frequent adjustments—I'm a big fan of trying something out for some time, and then making modifications if you're not making progress toward your goal. This has proved to be the most successful way for me to approach how I eat, and I think it's going to work great for you as well.

Eating for Your Best Results on The Turnaround

With that being said, the first adjustment I want you to make to your diet is *no adjustment at all.* You read that right. During the first two weeks of the plan, I want you to make *zero* changes to how you eat. What I do want you to do is simply eat as you normally eat, while keeping a detailed diary of what you eat and drink. Think of this as a low-pressure assignment to just start paying attention to your diet—although you will need to take this record keeping seriously because you're going to be relying on the information you gather later.

Here's what I want you to do:

1. Download any calorie-tracking app you like. I personally use MyFitnessPal because it's easy and allows me to scan food and build a library of the stuff I normally eat.

2. DO NOT CHANGE YOUR EATING HABITS (just in case you missed that the first time). For the first 14 days, I want you to simply input your food into the app (MyFitnessPal or others) and do it without skipping any snacks, meals, ice cream, drinks, etc. Yup, I want you to enter *everything* you eat into the app.

Like everything with The Turnaround, the key here is to complete this assignment while being totally honest with yourself. The goal of tracking your food without modifying your eating habits is to get a clear picture of your current diet—so lying, which is what you're doing if you eat something and don't record it, or cheating by inputting only half of what you ate will only give you a cloudy picture, and that's only going to hurt you in the long run. (Seriously, you'd only be cheating yourself—you'll see why in a minute.)

When I started tracking my food intake, it was the first time in my life that I could really see what I was putting into my body each day. And it helped me start to think a little about the choices I made that were just automatic, like always adding that second and third tablespoon of peanut butter to my PB&J. Come to find out, those tablespoons equaled about 250 unnecessary calories (do this daily for a year and that's basically over 180 meals of 500 empty calories each)—and yet, those sandwiches would have been just as good without the additional spoonfuls.

After two weeks of tracking, I want you to calculate your total caloric intake for the entire 14 days and then get the average daily intake.

HERE'S THE FORMULA: (Total sum of daily calories)/14 = average daily caloric intake

HERE'S AN EXAMPLE (your tally will have different numbers for each day, but you get the idea):

1,850 calories × 7 days = 12,950
2,000 calories × 7 days = 14,000
Total # of calories over all 14 days = 26,950
Total # of calories divided by 14 = 1,925 calories (26,950 ÷ 14 = 1,925)

Now, once you have your number, take a good look at it because this will be your calorie intake over the next three weeks. If your number was under 1,400 calories or over 2,000, I want you to make some adjustments:

IF YOUR DAILY AVERAGE IS UNDER 1,400 CALORIES: Put simply, if you are eating under 1,400 calories per day, then you're probably not eating enough food or you're a child. Bring your calories up to at least 1,400.

IF YOUR DAILY AVERAGE IS OVER 2,000 CALORIES: Unless you're secretly a performance athlete, you're probably eating too many empty calories—by empty calories, I mean "food" that has caloric count but little to no nutritional value. These are foods like Oreo cookies, Capri Sun, and my favorite: donuts (CRY FACE). Soooo, if your daily average is over 2,000 calories and you're looking to lose weight, then bring it down to 1,900 calories. But if you want to gain weight, then keep it as is but make sure to eat the whole foods you'll find on the shopping list.

Now, this is where things get really exciting because you aren't going to just eat for calories, you are going to eat for what's called *macros* and *micros*. If you've ever read any article on fitness, you've probably read about macros in one form or another. The mysterious "macros" is short for *macronutrients*, which are the nutrients that you need in large amounts (*macro* means large); these are protein, carbs, and fat. "Micros" (short for *micronutrients*) are trace elements like vitamins and fiber that your body needs in addition to macros. Please keep in mind that food doesn't have macros or micros in isolation—most foods provide a combination of protein, carbs, and fat. A little more about each:

PROTEIN: Proteins have four calories per gram and can be found in foods like chicken, beef, fish, pork, tempeh, and tofu. These foods go into the "protein" category because their ratio of protein compared to other macros is very high, but they might also contain some carbohydrates and/or fat. For example, a tuna steak, which is categorized as a protein, is 92% protein, 8% fat, and 0% carbs. Proteins are important to a number of functions in the body, including helping with structural development (e.g., muscle building) and chemical messaging that controls some hormones.

CARBS: Carbs also have four calories per gram and can be found in foods like vegetables, sweet potatoes, brown rice, and bread. Your body uses carbs, which are broken down into glucose, for energy. If you don't consume at least some carbs, your body will break down muscle to produce glucose. Complex and fibrous carbs are also very important to gut health, which rules your immune system.

FAT: Fats have nine calories per gram and include foods like peanut butter, olive oil, and avocado. Without healthy fat levels, your body essentially believes it's starving, and many bad things can happen. And guess what? You need some fat in your diet to be lean and mean. (More on this as we eat through this book.)

You'll want to familiarize yourself with these food categories because you'll start aiming to eat a certain percentage from each macro category every day. And P.S.: This isn't eating on another planet—your current diet already breaks out into certain macro percentages; you just don't know it because you haven't been paying attention. But you're awake now, remember? Creating progress requires next-level attention and choices made with intention.

How to Create Your Macros: Mel's 40-30-30 Approach

Once you have determined your daily caloric allowance, you are going to split it percentage-wise based on macros. My approach is to eat 40% carbs, 30% protein, and 30% fat. This is a split that allows for sustainability and results. Plus, it takes into consideration the realistic limits of what you can consume and what your body can actually break down and absorb. For example, you don't need to eat 200 grams of protein daily; that's waaaay overkill for most people, and it mostly just makes your digestive system work overtime for no added value. You will learn how to modify these percentages according to your goals as we move along.

Just so you know, if you're looking at this thinking *WTF, I have no idea how to do this* or *This biatch is speaking a foreign language*, that's totally normal and expected at this stage. But no need to worry—I'm going to walk you all the way through it. It'll just take a little bit of patience and, ahem, math. Sorry. It's all done in your best interest, I swear!! This is exactly how I learned to eat when I first started out, so I know it works!

What you want to do now is take your caloric intake and, using the macro percentages, determine how much of each you should be eating. Let's look at an example with a two-week average of 1,800 calories per day:

40% of these calories should be from carbs: 1,800 × 0.40 = 720 / 4 = 180 grams

30% of these calories should be from protein: 1,800 × .30 = 540 / 4 = 135 grams

30% of these calories should be from fat: 1,800 × 0.30 = 540 / 9 = 60 grams

These numbers—180 grams of carbs, 135 grams of protein, and 60 grams of fat—give you the real numbers that you'll need to pay attention to when you're figuring out what to eat. I know somebody out there just said, "HUH? What're you talking about, Mel? I don't see any *food* in there at all." Well, if you were to look up any food's nutritional value, you would see that its macros are broken down into grams. Here are a couple examples:

- A 5-ounce chicken breast would provide 43 grams of protein, 0 grams of carbs, and 5 grams of fat.

- A ½ cup serving of sweet potatoes would provide 1 gram of protein, 17 grams of carbs, and 4 grams of fat.

And all of these grams would count toward your macro totals for the day.

You can also see this type of information if you look at any packaged food with a label. For example, the label on a container of hummus might look like this:

Nutrition facts	Amount/serving	%DV*	Amount/serving	%DV*
Serv size 2 Tbsp (28g/1 oz)	Total Fat 5g	8%	Total Carb 4g	1%
Servings 7	Sat. Fat 1g	5%	Dietary Fiber 2g	8%
Calories 70	Trans Fat 0g		Sugars 0g	
Fat cal. 50	Cholest. 0mg	0%	Protein 2g	
*Percent Daily Values (DV) are	Sodium 130mg	5%		
Based on 2,000 calorie diet.	Vitamin A 0% • Vitamin C 0% • Calcium 2% • Iron 4 %			

So, if you had one serving of two tablespoons, this would add 4 grams of carbs, 2 grams of protein, and 5 grams of fat to your macros. Now, a lot of the stuff you'll be eating on The Turnaround won't have a label (in fact, that's how you know you're eating the best stuff for your body!), which is why you'll have to rely on a tracking app to tell you the macro info.

Here's the great news: If your brain is exploding a little or you don't want to do all this work, plenty of food tracking apps will do more than just tell you the macro info—they'll actually allow you to set your macros and automatically count up the totals for you. But I still seriously hope you'll take the time to understand the math because it will help you connect more with what you're eating. Some people find that eating for macros gives them, for the first time, a trackable structure that leaves no room for confusion over what they should be eating. For others, macros free them from the straitjacket of a pure calorie-based approach to eating. Ultimately, I think macros represent a gateway into understanding the components of food in a new way.

The Nutrition "Catch"

If you've heard about macros, you might have also heard that people think that all you've gotta do is eat based on these percentages and you're good. Meaning that you can eat whatever crap foods you want, and it doesn't matter as long as you've met your macros. That's not how it's gonna work on The Turnaround. There's a catch to eating for your macros Mel-style: I want you to get all your calories, every single day, from nutrient-rich foods (those label-free foods I was talking about).

The reason for this is that not all calories are created equal; some are trash calories that really don't do much for your body. Sure, your cells will metabolize trash calories, but they'll still be hungry for more, hungry for the quality goods they can use to build that dreamy body you desire. Luckily for you, I have included all the nutrition-based recipes and guidelines you need, and I'm going to help you discover that nutrition-packed foods don't have to be dull, bland, and boring.

"Are My Macros Working?": When to Check In on Your Progress

During this first rotation, you're going to make adjustments as you work to dial in your nutrition to make sure it's just right for you. Here's when to check in on things (I'll remind you when it's time to do this in the weekly calendar coming up at the end of this chapter):

AT THE START OF WEEK 6: After three weeks of eating a nutrition-based diet and sticking to your macros, it will be time to do a quick check-in on how it's working for you, making adjustments as needed.

If you started losing weight, I want you to add another 100 calories to your daily intake and split them evenly across carbs and fat, but do not up your protein intake. So, if your daily allowance was 1,800 calories and you lost a few pounds in the last few weeks, then add another 100 calories to your daily intake in the form of 50 calories (12g) from carbs and 50 calories (6g) from fat.

I know what you're thinking: "You want me to add calories if I'm losing? But my goal is to *lose* weight?!" Well, *my* goal is to move you toward a sustainable caloric intake, which is why I want you to creep the calories up a little if what you're doing is working. If you are eating a nutrition-focused diet, your body will adjust and continue losing unneeded fat while supporting muscle growth and proper functioning. By moving your body toward a sustainable intake, you can enjoy the benefits of long-term weight loss and say goodbye to gaining-losing-gaining every time you change something in your diet or go on vacation. Remember, our goal is to have a sexy but healthy body 4eva.

Here's an example of your new intake (1,900 calories):

Daily carbs: 192g
Daily protein: 135g (stayed the same)
Daily fat: 66g

The End of Undereating

If you're coming to this from an outdated "eating less = weight loss" mindset, I want you to know it's not cute or cool to undereat on The Turnaround. (Don't think I don't know that you're going to try to be all sneaky with yourself—remember, I've been where you are now! You can't hide nothin' from me.) I know how crazy-hard it is to override this instinct, because you've been programmed to think that *not* feeding your body will give you the body you want. This. Doesn't. Work. Trust me. Turn your efforts instead to working on hitting your numbers, your carb, fat, and protein targets. I'd even rather you go slightly over than under these goals. If you see that you're a little short on your macros, use the Nutrient-Rich Sides section in the Recipes chapter (page 143) to make sure you can get those 10 grams of carbs you may have missed on your daily intake.

If you haven't lost any weight at the Week 6 check-in, DO NOTHING. Yes, do nothing—your body needs more time to move to a healthy metabolic state. I know this sounds crazy, but your body loses unneeded weight at a healthy rate when it's nourished, not when it's forced into a controlled starvation of sorts.

10 Days Later—and Then, 10 Days After That

Ten days after your Week 6 check-in, weigh yourself and take your measurements—sometimes you will see your weight stay the same, but your body will literally look and measure dramatically different. Based on your results, use the same protocol explained above: If you lost weight, up your carbs and fat intake by 100 calories. No changes = do nothing. I recommend continuing with this schedule of checking in on your progress every 10 days. In the calendar, watch for the ✎ symbol in the Mouth blurbs that open each week. The ✎ symbol will indicate a 10-day check-in is coming up during that week and tell you what day it should fall on.

"Will I Count Macros Until the End of Time?"

So, once you're at that 2,000 to 2,500 daily caloric intake of a nutrition-based diet, you have been training consistently in the gym and feel you have a good hang on the exercises (this will happen generally after 12 to 16 weeks on the program), and you also look and feel healthy and strong, then you may decide not to track macros or do your check-in every 10 days. Yup, you can let go of tracking and calculations and listen to your body, since now you have nutritional and training intuition. All that training is so your body can do the work and your mind won't be too occupied with the details of your pursuit; this will open the door to the higher pursuits in your life such as career, family, and taking over the world.

It's About Patience, Not Perfection

The Turnaround is a six-month program for a reason: because a legitimate body transformation takes at least that long. Other programs that try to sell you on a 30-day miracle are lying! Sure, you can make a difference in 30 days, but there's no transformation happening in that time frame, no matter who you are. A big part of this is because it usually takes about 3 to 6 months to find the ideal caloric/nutritional intake for *you*, as I mentioned above. This ideal depends upon so much—your activity level, age, genetics, hormones, etc. What's crazy is that some of these factors change every day, so your ideal can even vary day to day—but trust me: With patience, you will zero in on a general zone that can ride out the bumpy, bluesy, and downright bad days.

What you can focus on as your nutrition and metabolism get sorted out is continuing to deepen your understanding of food. The more you know, the less attention you have to pay down the road—you just start to automatically know how many carbs work best for you or what kind of protein makes you feel the leanest. Pretty soon you're gonna have some kind of X-ray vision that allows you to impress your friends: "You see that piece of steak? That's got xx grams of protein and xx grams of fat." Okay, no one's really going to be impressed by this—you may even get a bit annoying with this at first, LOL—but because you are going to look so freakin' bangin', they will at least pretend to listen for a minute.

Again, the goal is for you to allow your body to settle, eat the best nutrition-based foods possible, understand how your body works on food, develop a better relationship with food, and ultimately keep moving toward being the person you want to be from the inside out—and yes, have visible abs! Okay, that was more like six goals instead of one, but my point is that I want you never to stray too far from the fact that every effort, every little extra bit of attention that you squeeze out of yourself is going to pay you back—it's *all* an investment in you.

Keep in mind that when you're around the intake of 2,000 to 2,500 daily nutritional calories per day, your body is either at or moving toward its ideal weight. (Again: Pay attention to how you feel and look, health indicators, etc., and not to an arbitrary number in your head, like "125 pounds.") As you progress through this program, I guarantee that you'll move from obsessing over numbers to understanding how your body moves and feels at different intakes. The process of figuring out what to eat and how much will be *intuitive*.

The Turnaround Shopping List

After you go through your two weeks of tracking what you eat without making changes, then it's time to figure your macros and start cooking closer to a nutrition-based approach—aka it's time to go to the supermarket and make some of my recipes!

The list below is meant to help you figure out what to buy and cook, even if you don't follow my recipes exactly. Yup, if you don't like venison, for example, just replace it with tempeh or chicken or whatever you like from the list. You can find 90% or more of these items at your local Trader Joe's, Whole Foods, Kroger, etc. I know this because this is the same list I use all the time—the foods I've made my recipes from for years.

Proteins	Carbs	Seasonings
Beef (96/4 fat ratio)	Brown rice	Fresh garlic
Venison	White rice	Onions
Bison	Sweet potatoes	Paprika
Chicken	Red potatoes	Oregano
(antibiotic free/organic)	Multigrain bread	Crushed red pepper
Salmon	Couscous	Black pepper
Tuna	Quinoa	Sea salt
Cod	Beans	
Eggs	Steel-cut oats	
Turkey		
Plain Greek yogurt		
Shrimp		
Red snapper		
Tofu		

Nuts
Cashews
Almonds
Pistachios
Granola
Chia seeds

Fruits
Avocado
Bananas
Apples
Blackberries
Blueberries
Raspberries
Strawberries
Coconut

Oils
Coconut oil
Olive oil
Sunflower oil

Condiments
Hot sauce
Mustard
Tabasco sauce

Dressings
Olive oil
Apple cider vinegar
Balsamic vinegar

Veggies
Broccoli rabe
Broccolini
Cauliflower
Brussels sprouts
Kale
Edamame
Baby spinach
Zucchini
Green beans
Black beans
Carrots
Peas
Peppers (any)
Broccoli
Asparagus
Eggplant

Drinks
Water
Coffee
Herbal tea
Unsweetened almond milk

Supplements (Optional)
Fish oil
Probiotic
Digestive enzymes
Vitamin A
Vitamin C
Vitamin D

A Couple Categories That Deserve Special Attention

Some additional thoughts on a couple sneaky-ass "food" categories that can mess with your metabolism. These are 1) beverages and 2) sugary or synthetic crapstuff. You gotta really watch out for the crapstuff because it will do nada, nothing, zip for you and your goals.

Beverages

Listen up: You're about to become real tight with a little hottie known as H_2O. I want you to gaze into that clear, cleansing, calorie-free source of hydration like you are in love with it and everything it's going to do for you. Water helps flush waste, hydrate skin, lubricate joints, regulate mood, increase metabolism—it's so good for you that I want you to aim to drink a gallon of it every single day. Yes, I said a gallon—128 ounces of water every damn day. No complaints. Get yourself a reusable bottle and fill that thing up every chance you get. Once you start drinking it consistently throughout the day, you'll notice that you actually feel thirstier, and this will make it easier to keep grabbing for that bottle. Yes, this means you'll be going to the bathroom a lot!

Besides water, you can drink coffee and tea as long as they're not supersize, more-sugar-than-caffeine-uccinos. If you're drinking caffeinated varieties, lean toward moderation because you will absolutely need quality sleep to help you recover, and caffeine and sleep do not mix. Try to keep your caffeine intake to one or two cups per day, no more than that—well, maybe three cups on those days that you feel like you won't survive without a little jolt of coffee juice in the afternoon. If you want to chill with some tea at night, go with a nice, calming option—you know, one of those that have goofy-looking bears in pajamas on it—so you don't stare at the fucking ceiling all night. (If you're like me, it's not caffeine, but your crazy head that keeps you up at night. But that's for another chapter!)

Sugar, Sweeteners, and Synthetic Foods

See also dried fruits, sauces, fat-free, sugar-free, zero-calorie trail mix, protein cookies, and so on.

The short answer is NO to all that. The food-marketing industry likes to call these products different names, but they are all the same: food-like items that contain no nutritional value and do not contribute anything to your health and well-being. Fruit is okay as long as you eat the ones that have a decent amount of fiber. Fake sweeteners and chemical additives play tricks on your taste buds and on appetite hormones, and they just confuse the shit out of your body. Stay away from them as much as possible.

MUSCLE

So, what kinds of workouts can you expect to help you build that body of your dreams? I have designed the entire program to get you off the couch and into the gym, which means the workouts are progressive and speak to the increases in strength and skill you will experience as you make your way through the program.

There are two main categories of workouts with different subcategories: bodyweight workouts and gym/equipment-based workouts:

BODYWEIGHT WORKOUTS. These will be high-intensity interval training, or HIIT, workouts. You won't need anything more than your body for these (no equipment!), so you can do them at home. But don't be fooled into thinking that this makes them easy. Oh, no, no, no—not even close, my dear. The HIIT workouts are the most intense and rewarding 20-minute workouts you can imagine, and they only get more fun as you get stronger.

You will find the bodyweight workouts in the first rotation, where we want to 1) focus on developing your neuromuscular response (nerves plus muscles working together), 2) send a seriously strong message to any unneeded fat that we are coming for you, and 3) lay the base layer for some structurally sound muscles.

GYM WORKOUTS. You will need to go to the gym to do these equipment-based workouts. You will be lifting weights to develop aesthetically attractive muscles that are strong and flexible, and will help you move in ways you never thought possible. This development will form the foundation for any demanding physical activity, inside and outside of the gym, that you may perform in the future. You will learn all the fundamental lifts—squats, dead lifts, presses, rows—and the mechanically correct way to perform them for your body— that is, without pain or injury. There will be load progressions (using different sets and reps to push your strength and performance), core and athletic performance development exercises, explosiveness, and a ton of fun packed into your lifting experience with me!

You will find that the program is designed around ranges of sets (a block containing reps) and reps (number of repetitions for a move), such as "4 sets of 12–15 reps" or "4 × 12–15" for short. This means that you will perform that particular move 12 to 15 times for 4 sets, which will give you a total of 48 to 60 reps.

Let's say that your exercise asks for this: "Squats: 7 × 10"

This means that you will do 7 sets of 10 reps of squats (for 70 total squats). Simple, right? And it is—there will be no calculus required to figure out my workouts, I promise!

Or perhaps the exercise looks like this: "Mountain climbers: 3 × 30 seconds"

This means that you will do 3 sets of mountain climbers for 30 seconds per set.

Of course, the other essential factor is how much weight you should lift. This is probably one of the most important elements to making progress in the gym. The only element that should come before the matter of your weight selection is form. So, your mission, should you choose to accept it, is to:

First, work *really* hard on learning to do every exercise with the best form possible. I want you to come into the gym every day with the mentality that you're learning everything for the first time ever; this approach will keep you improving and healthy, and it will keep the ego in check.

Next, you will want to lift the *heaviest* weights or create the *greatest* resistance possible while maintaining the *best* form possible. And this applies to both women and men; it makes no difference!

Here's how to check if you're lifting the heaviest weights possible: If your set calls for 10 reps and you do all of them without feeling challenged, then you're lifting too light. On the next set, go heavier. Your goal is to barely make it through those 10 reps while struggling to get there—this should take TONS of focus and concentration. I want you to challenge yourself, even if it means constantly changing the weight you lift.

If you're wondering if there will be any rest included in your workouts, the answer is yes, *sometimes*. Unless stated otherwise for a particular workout, you should keep moving to the next exercise as soon as you're done with your sets; don't take more than 45 seconds to about 1 minute of rest between sets. I recommend that you ignore your phone and outside distractions at all costs—this is your time, and your complete focus will pay off.

And before you move into the first rotation, I'll address the burning-hot question of abs—*Will I see them???* Well, The Turn-

Ladies Who Lift

Ladies: You won't turn into a man because you lift weights or because you lift heavy weights—that's not how your body works, biologically. Women with extremely developed muscles got there from sources other than lifting alone, or they are women who have made their bodies their job.

around is designed to help you build a really strong core, which will help create killer abs (which I'm sorry to say will not be visible until you're on point with your nutrition for at least 6 to 12 weeks, depending on your starting position). That is, if you are 10 pounds off your ideal weight, you will get visible abs (and a bangin' booty!) much faster than if you're 100 pounds off.

THE TURNAROUND 45°: WEEKS 1–8 CALENDAR

Week 1

Mouth

 Pop Quiz: You should be ready to make a gazillion changes to your diet today. True or False?

FALSE. I don't want you to make any changes right now. But I do want you to keep track of what you're eating and drinking this week and next, as I explained in the previous section on food and macros (page 58). This means documenting enough information about your daily diet so that you can use it later to calculate your caloric intake.

Mind

 When I first started working out 6-plus years ago, do you think I knew what I was doing?! I was so clueless. I had all the same questions you probably have now:

1. How do I get started?
2. Where do I get motivation?
3. Will I ever look like *that*?
4. How long does it take?
5. Am I doing enough?
6. What the fuck do I eat, and how much?
7. Can I really do this?
8. What if I don't make any changes?
9. How am I going to fit all this into my day?
10. It's so much info—how will I learn everything?

It's like learning how to drive: When you first get in the car you're like, "How the fuck am I gonna look at all these mirrors and the road and move my feet and turn the wheel and stay in the lane all at the same time? LOL. (Now, this is coming from a girl who learned how to drive at 32 years old.) But somehow you just get it and it becomes natural.

I promise that all your questions will be answered, *but only* if you *do* it every day, do something that is in line with the person you want to be, with the person you already *are* underneath all the bullshit you tell yourself. You are there! Just believe!

Muscle

 ### Day One: Legs & Abs

In-and-out abs: 3 × 30 seconds (take 30 seconds' rest between sets)

High knees: 3 × 30 seconds (take 30 seconds' rest between sets)

Banded hamstring curls: 3 × 100

Hamstring curl machine: 5 × 20 (As you move through the sets, be sure to increase the load and challenge yourself while staying within the rep range)

Dead lifts: 4 × 12–15

Squats (bodyweight): 4 × 15–20

Adductor machine: 4 × 20

Mel's Tip

Banded work and bodywork are the best way to target specific muscles and get some nice blood flow so your workout can be efficient AF!

Day Two: Upper-Body Hybrid

Banded straight-arm pull-downs: 3 × 60

Lat pull-downs (wide grip): 4 × 15

Bent-over rear delt barbell rows: 4 × 12–15

Biceps straight-bar curls: 5 × 15–20

Biceps E-Z bar curls: 5 × 12–15

Triceps cable push-downs (straight bar): 5 × 15–20

E-Z bar skull crushers on bench: 5 × 10–15

When you're doing bent-over rows, you want to sit into your hips, which means your butt cheeks should be tight AF. And when pulling the bar toward the top of your belly button, think of your elbows moving toward the ceiling and pushing your chest out as you pull, so your shoulders don't cave in.

Day Three: Cardio

Stairmaster: 25 minutes at steady speed (I like 6.0)

Take 45–60 seconds between sets on the next exercises:

High knees: 4 × 30 seconds

Hip thrusts (Smith machine): 4 × 20

Kick-backs (bodyweight): 5 × 20 (each leg)

Day Four: Chest & Triceps & Shoulders

Smith machine flat chest presses: 4 × 15–20

Dumbbell incline chest presses: 4 × 12–15

Triceps dips using bodyweight (bench): 4 × 20

Triceps cable push-downs (straight bar): 5 × 12–15

Standing rope triceps pull-overs: 4 × 12–15

Shoulder presses (banded): 4 × 50

Military presses: 4 × 12–15

Mouth: Follow-Up

If I had time, I'd start a #savethecarbs campaign. Seriously. Carbohydrates are not the devil. I mean, shitty, processed carbs are pretty damn bad for you—at best, a waste of calories, at worst, the number one reason the world is facing a type-2 diabetes epidemic. So, maybe those types of carbs could fall under the devilish category. And by shitty, processed carbs, I'm talking about chips, cookies, candy bars, and most boxed or packaged foods. But you go on and eat whatever you want for one more week. I'm not trying to influence your choices. Nope. Not one bit.

Week 2

Mouth

Another week of eating whatever the hell you want (enjoy it while it lasts!), but keep tracking every detail. And now's a good time for a hydration check: How's your water intake? Do you have to pee every 10 minutes? If so, you're good. I'm exaggerating a little—but not much.

If you haven't obtained a refillable water bottle, be sure to track one down. And if you're broke as shit (been there) and all you can afford is a value pack of water from Walmart, that is all you fucking need. To stay hydrated, you don't *need* a fancy $70 steel bottle that can survive Armageddon. Just get whatever you can and carry it with you at all times, refilling it whenever you can. Check out the Tap app to find out where you can refill your water bottle based on your location.

Mel's Tip

I recommend glass or high-grade aluminum bottles—I know glass is a dangerous proposition, but you can get one with a silicone cover—because plastics, even BPA-free or whatever, behave in chemically questionable ways and are even affected by temperature. Even a "safe" plastic bottle can become dangerous if it's left out in the sun all day.

Mind

It's become harder for me to respond to every DM on Instagram, but some of them stand out—one chica sent me this message: "Mel, how can I lose weight really fast?" Heh. Well, I'm glad you asked because it's super-duper easy, like you just stare at your body in the mirror really hard and pretty soon your weight will just fall off like leaves from a tree. (Just kidding—I tried that for years and never could get it to work.)

Here's how I really replied to this person: *You can start by not asking lazy questions.* Oops. That might have been a little harsh. But it's the truth! What I've learned is this: What you get fast you lose even faster. All good things take time and patience and if you're not willing to go hard, I suggest you go home. How's that for a warm welcome to Week 2? You've got this.

Muscle

Day One: Legs & Abs

Alternating knees to elbows: 3 × 10 (touching each knee to elbow once is 1 rep; take 30-second rest)

Squats (bodyweight): 5 × 30, 20, 15, 12, 20 (first set is 30 reps, second is 20—last set is 20 reps)

Dead lifts: 5 × 30, 20, 15, 12, 20

Hamstring extension machine: 4 × 20 (as you move through the sets, be sure to increase the load and challenge yourself while staying within the rep range)

Quad extension machine: 4 × 20

Sumo squats with dumbbells: 5 × 30, 20, 15, 12, 20

Day Two: Cardio

PART 1 *(start with 70% resistance and increase by 10% every week)*

Stairmaster: 25 minutes at steady speed

PART 2

Jump rope: 3 sets, 100 jumps (take 30 seconds' rest between sets)

Hip thrusts (Smith machine): 4 × 20

Air squats: 4 × 30

Day Three: Upper-Body Hybrid

Biceps E-Z bar curls: 4 × 15–20

Alternating biceps dumbbell curls: 4 × 10–12 (each arm)

Standing rope triceps pull-overs: 4 × 15–20

Triceps cable push-downs (straight bar): 4 × 12–15

Military presses: 4 × 15–20

Seated shoulder presses: 4 × 12–15

Day Four: Cardio & Abs

LISS (low-intensity steady-state treadmill walk): 25 minutes at 2.8 speed/8.0 incline

Kneeling rope crunches: 4 × 20

Lying leg lifts: 4 × 20

In-and-out abs: 3 × 30 seconds (take 30 seconds' rest between sets)

Get jiggy in the gym, even just for a moment. Shake it out—stop gripping the weights so damn tight. Remember to have fun (after or in between crushing it). Of course, you can use emotion and anger to power your workouts at first, but soon that'll dissipate, and you'll be left with nada. Instead of drawing on any anger or problems, have some fun. Don't take this shit too seriously—let your body produce results that you can enjoy, cuz they're coming from fun. You don't want no angry abs, girl.

Mouth: Follow-Up

We took the veil down from your food intake during these past two weeks; you were able to discover your eating habits, and how often you were really going to the cookie jar or the secret candy stash in your nightstand drawer. Like me, you may have realized you lied to yourself a ton because you ate empty calories and then didn't want to enter it into the app because you knew exactly what you were doing.

Your brain is going to start looking for all the things you should have done differently, you will punish yourself for all the bad choices, and you will try to stress over food as you usually do. *STOP.* The goal is to be honest, but to be compassionate, to make meaningful choices and take action—all the mental chatter doesn't help decision-making, so let it go as much as you can. Take where you are right now and accept it as a transition to where you want to be; nothing more than that.

Remember, at this point it's time to add up your caloric intake over the last two weeks to get your average, which is your calorie goal for the next three weeks (21 days). Jump back to page 59 for how to calculate your average.

Week 3

Mouth

At this stage in the journey, you've got your calorie goal and you're ready to start eating right. So, what do you eat? Right now, you need easy and good and consistent. (Yes, that means eating the same dish for every breakfast, another dish for every lunch, and another dish for every dinner this week.) I suggest starting with three dishes that are easy to make and easy to take along with you, if needed. I personally would go with these three (they can be found in the recipes section):

Meal 1: Huevos Rancheros + Baby Spinach
Meal 2: Flank Steak with Sautéed Zucchini + Cauliflower
Meal 3: Brown Rice Poke Bowl

Mind

 Sitting through the discomfort of change is DISCIPLINE.
Sticking to your word through the process is STRENGTH.
Doing this day in and day out is LOVE.
It seems worse before it gets better is TRUTH.

You've made the decision to get to where you are, and you're exactly where you need to be.
Are you ready to get uncomfortable? Speak your shit into existence!

Muscle

 Day One: Upper-Body Hybrid
Smith machine flat chest presses: 4 × 30, 20, 15, 20 (first set is 30 reps, second set is 20 reps, third set 15 reps, last set is 20 reps)
Dumbbell incline chest presses: 4 × 12–15
Seated V-bar cable rows: 4 × 30, 20, 15, 20
Lat pull-downs (wide grip): 4 × 12–15
Lat pull-downs (supinated narrow grip): 4 × 12–15
Biceps straight-bar curls: 4 × 15
Alternating biceps dumbbell curls: 4 × 12 each arm

Day Two: Cardio
Stairmaster: 25 minutes at steady speed (6.0)
Take 45–60 seconds between sets on the next exercises:
Hip thrusts (Smith machine): 4 × 20
Drop squats (banded): 30
Mountain climbers: 3 × 30 seconds

Engaging Your Back Muscles 101

1. Know where your back muscles are (see page 42).

2. Focus and feel the muscle you're working when in motion. You can practice this with a super light weight or no weight at all.

3. Shoulders back and away from your ears, chest up! (THIS IS THE MOST IMPORTANT.)

4. When pulling, think of where your elbows are, point them in the direction you want to go, and think of them moving in that direction. Your hands no longer exist; they are now part of the mechanism you're using.

5. Push your chest forward as you pull your elbows down or behind you (THIS IS A BIG ONE).

6. Push ring and pinky fingers into the bar and make sure your palm is touching the bar as well (GET A GOOD GRIP!).

   NOW: Do all these things at once and your *whole life* will change.

Day Three: Legs & Abs
Kneeling rope crunches: 4 × 20
Lying leg lifts: 3 × 20
Scissors: 3 × 20 (each leg)
Squats (bodyweight): 4 × 10–15
Goblet squats: 4 × 10–12
Hamstring curl machine: 4 × 20
Adductor machine: 4 × 20

Day Four: Upper-Body Hybrid

Seated V-bar cable rows: 4 × 12–15

Lat V-bar pull-downs: 4 × 10–12

Lat pull-downs (wide grip): 4 × 10–12

Standing rope triceps pull-overs: 4 × 15–20

Assisted dips: 4 × 10–15

Seated Smith machine shoulder presses: 4 × 15–20

Arnold presses: 4 × 10–12

.... *Mel's Tip* ....

Think of your workout as a form of movement meditation. *Be* the focus. Remove everything else.

Mouth: Follow-Up

So, you're probably wondering which carbs I would save as part of my #savethecarbs campaign. I would definitely defend the real, whole-foods type of carbohydrates like sweet potatoes, whole-grain bread, brown rice, quinoa, steel-cut oats, beans, and most vegetables as having a solid place in a healthy diet. Your body will be eager to metabolize the nutrients found in these carbs, using what's needed immediately and storing the rest as glycogen in your tissues for later energy demands. These types of carbohydrates are especially good after you've hit the weights extra hard.

Week 4

Mouth

If you still have moments where you wonder *Should I eat this?* I have one simple rule I like to follow: If it doesn't grow in the soil (I've wished more than once that there were cake trees, LOL), don't eat it.

Oh, and if you're wondering what to eat every day this week, give the sample menu below a try, but this week feel free to swap in some of the recipes from last week if you preferred those. You're building a nutrient-rich menu one recipe and meal at a time.

Meal 1: Strawberry Banana smoothie

Meal 2: Beef and Broccoli + White Rice

Meal 3: Salmon + Sweet Potatoes + Asparagus
Meal 4: Bibimbap + Baby Spinach

You may have noticed that I went from three meals a day to four here. In my personal experience, three to four meals seems to hit home and allows me the portion size plus variety combination I enjoy. You may choose to try it or stick with three meals a day.

Mind

Right about now, you might start noticing your mind getting a little twitchy, talking a little smack—saying things like, "I've been working my ass off, why don't I look like the Instagram fit chicks already?!! What the hell are they doing that I'm not?!" And I'll tell you something—I asked myself these questions over and over the *first two years* of consistently eating right and training hard. What I didn't know or what I didn't want to believe was that these chicks had years of hard work behind them, and not just one or two years, more like between five and 10 years of being *consistently* dedicated.

I'm not saying it's going to take you that long to hit your goal, but I am trying to help you get real with your expectations because I didn't really get it until I was on the inside—and now I'm reporting back to you with intel.

If you've been putting in the work and really truly doing your best, then the only thing you're missing is time. Keep on keepin' on! I was 200 pounds once with pretty much zero muscle—think about that.

Muscle

Day One: Legs & Abs
Lying leg lifts: 3 × 20
Scissors: 3 × 20 (each leg)
Mountain climbers: 3 × 30 seconds (take 30 seconds' rest between sets)
Dead lifts: 4 × 10–12
Leg presses (wide stance): 4 × 10–15
Hamstring extension machine: 4 × 20
Adductor machine: 4 × 20

Day Two: Movement Hybrid

Stairmaster: 25 minutes at steady speed

Military presses: 4 × 10–15

Plyo split lunges: 4 × 10 (each leg)

Drop squats (banded): 4 × 20

KB (kettlebell) swings: 4 × 40 (find a weight that challenges you!)

Lying leg lifts: 4 × 20

Jump rope: 5 minutes

Day Three: Upper Body

Seated V-bar cable rows: 4 × 12–15

Lat pull-downs (wide grip): 4 × 12–15

Bent-over dumbbell rows: 4 × 10 (together)

Biceps straight-bar curls: 4 × 20

Biceps barbell curls: 4 × 12–15

Barbell preacher curls: 4 × 12–15

Day Four: Legs & Shoulders

Squats (wide stance): 4 × 10–15

Leg presses: 4 × 10

Quad extension machine: 4 × 20

Hamstring curl machine: 5 × 20

Seated calf raises: 4 × 10–15

Military presses: 4 × 20

Arnold presses: 4 × 20

Lateral raises: 4 × 15–20

Mouth: Follow-Up

So the first two weeks you ate whatever you wanted. And then these past two weeks you've followed my meal plan suggestions to perfection. Well, headed into week 5 I want you to know you don't need to overthink this. If you want to just eat rice, chicken, sweet potatoes, and veggies arranged differently for all your meals, then do it. Buy a rice maker and make either white or brown rice, choose different veggie recipes, and then boil some Japanese sweet potatoes (I like their texture better) and put your meals in glass containers. This technique won't last you long, but you can go with it for one to two weeks until you sort out how to allocate your time. Point is, don't stress.

Week 5

Mouth

Are you eating enough food? You shouldn't think of yourself as dieting while on The Turnaround. Yes, you are following a specific diet, but you should absolutely not be starving yourself and eating just a bunch of salads and shitty, zero-calorie or sugar-free drinks. A changing body needs to be fed; a working body is hungry as hell for nutrition—be sure you're giving those muscles what they need! Eat some vegetables, grains, eggs, potatoes, fruits, fish, chicken—enjoy all the good stuff, the really good stuff, not the fluff and filler that you used to think was the good stuff.

Mel's Tip

Don't accept laziness from yourself; a protein bar is not lunch. Keep preppin' and packin' (lunch, silly), or find a trustworthy spot where you can pick up some simple, tasty, and healthy food. For example, find a local Mediterranean restaurant and ask for roasted chicken (or whichever is the simplest chicken they have) plus grilled veggies without any butter or oil, and ask if they have some plain rice or pasta. Done.

Mind

You might feel a little dip in motivation right about now, or it might hit you next week. Either way, there will be this little voice in you that starts talking shit about quitting. Don't listen to that whiny B; she's the same one who tried to use anger and emotion at the beginning because she knows those don't last. Hold on for just a bit longer and you'll be rewarded with an unexpected wave of momentum. Get ready to ride that shit—it's coming!!

Muscle

Day One: Legs & Abs
Kneeling rope crunches: 4 × 20
Lying leg lifts: 4 × 20
Plank hold: 4 × 1 minute
Banded diagonal-forward crab walks: 3 × 10 (each leg)
Squats (bodyweight): 5 × 10
Dead lifts: 5 × 10
Hamstring extension machine: 4 × 20
Quad extension machine: 4 × 20

Day Two: Back & Biceps
Biceps rope curls: 5 × 20
Biceps E-Z bar curls: 5 × 12–15
Alternating biceps dumbbell curls: 4 × 10
Cable rows: 4 × 12–15
Lat pull-downs (wide grip): 4 × 12–15
Lat pull-downs (supinated narrow grip): 4 × 8–12
Bent-over dumbbell rows: 4 × 10 (together)
Pull-ups (band assisted): 3 × 10

Day Three: Cardio
Stairmaster: 30 minutes at steady speed (6.0)
Take 45–60 seconds between sets on the next exercises:
High knees: 5 × 30 seconds
Drop squats (banded): 20 reps
Mountain climbers: 3 × 30 seconds

Day Four: Chest & Triceps & Shoulders
Cable chest flies: 4 × 20
Barbell flat chest presses: 4 × 12–15
Dumbbell incline chest presses: 4 × 12–15
Triceps cable push-downs (straight bar): 5 × 20

Skull crushers (incline bench and dumbbells): 4 × 20

Assisted dips: 4 × 10–15

Military presses: 4 × 10–15

Dumbbell flat chest presses: 4 × 10

Mouth: Follow-Up

Headed into week 6, with all the freedom in the world to create your own nutrient-rich meal plan, this is a great opportunity for you to try using the stand-alone recipes for micros, carbs, and proteins! I wrote them so that you'll know how to make certain staples for you and your family, and to help you learn to cook an array of different dishes that can be combined into dozens of recipes. Here's a sample:

Meal 1: Fried Eggs + Sweet Potatoes + Baby Spinach

Meal 2: Beef + White Rice + Asparagus

Meal 3: Chicken + Brown Rice + Kale

Meal 4: Salmon + Eggplant + Broccoli

Week 6

Mouth

You've been eating based on your customized caloric intake for three weeks at this point. Now, it's time to make an adjustment based on your progress. If you are making progress toward your goal, then you can add those 100 calories split evenly between carbs and fat. If you are trying to lose weight and your results seem slow or stalled, I want you to take a deep breath and relax, then leave everything the same and give your body another 10 days to settle metabolically.

Mind

People always say things like "I wish I had your confidence." I didn't always have confidence, but when you work so fucking hard for something, like really, really do your best to master it, you feel proud and empowered and no one can take that from you EVER!

Real, rooted, unshakable confidence doesn't come from nothing; you've got to create it. You create it by first focusing on YOU rather than getting caught up comparing yourself to other people. Then, you identify your goals and put them in front of you and start putting in the work. You put in the work until suddenly you start to feel like you're in control—that's your confidence breaking through. Be consistent with the work and your sense of control will strengthen, and with it your confidence.

Of course, the first steps can feel scary, but if you've identified a goal, that means you've identified something you want, even need, in your life—and that something can be yours. Do the work over and over until you gain mastery. Confidence doesn't come from magic; it comes from practice.

Muscle

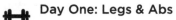 Day One: Legs & Abs

Lying leg lifts: 4 × 20

Jumping jacks: 3 × 20

Squats (bodyweight): 5 × 30, 20, 15, 12, 20

Dead lifts: 5 × 30, 20, 15, 12, 20

Dumbbell stiff-leg dead lifts: 4 × 10–12

Hamstring curl machine: 5 × 20

Quad extension machine: 4 × 20

Kneeling rope crunches: 5 × 20–30

Day Two: Cardio

Stairmaster: 25 minutes at steady speed

Jump rope: 4 × 60 seconds

Mountain climbers: 3 × 30 seconds (take 30 seconds' rest between sets)

Day Three: Upper-Body Hybrid

Biceps rope curls: 4 × 20

Biceps E-Z bar curls: 4 × 12–15

Alternating biceps dumbbell curls: 4 × 10–12

Triceps cable pull-downs (rope): 4 × 20

Seated triceps pull-overs: 4 × 15–20

Shoulder presses with barbell: 4 × 15–20

Seated shoulder presses: 4 × 12–15

Day Four: Cardio & Abs

LISS (treadmill walk): 25 minutes at 4.0 speed/5.0 incline

Bicycle sprints: 10 minutes (alternate 15 seconds' sprinting with 45 seconds at a normal pace for 10 minutes)

Kneeling rope crunches: 4 × 20

Lying leg lifts: 4 × 20

Scissors: 4 × 20 (each leg)

Mel's Tip

Low-intensity steady-state cardio, aka LISS cardio, is a way to burn calories without over-elevating your heart rate or increasing your cardiovascular output. We do this to push your cells slowly toward using any stored fat, and to burn calories without tapping into your body's glycogen reserves. When the weather is nice, I like going on a 45-minute walk outside (look for something with an incline!) instead of walking on a treadmill.

Mouth: Follow-Up

It may not be nutritionally necessary, but I'm pretty fucking sure I would not survive without coffee. I don't know what I need more: the caffeine or the morning ritual of making coffee—it's probably a tie.

Have you created a morning ritual, whether it's making coffee or tea for yourself or reading 10 pages of a book? I think of this time as providing a different sort of nourishment than food—it nourishes this place of peace inside me that I know is there, but it needs a little attention *from me* to come to life. It doesn't respond to love from others; this peace has gotta be self-grown, baby. Be sure to carve out this time—not a single second of it will ever feel wasted!

Week 7

Mouth

When you hit day three of this week—which will be 10 days of eating at your customized caloric intake—check your progress. Then, adjust the same as before: If you're losing weight, add 100 calories split evenly between carbs and fat. If you're not losing weight, do nothing. If you want to gain weight and nothing is happening, again, add 100 calories split evenly between carbs and fat. Be consistent for the next 10 days after that ("day one" will start the day *after* your check-in) so you can make realistic adjustments based on disciplined eating.

 Get your 10-day check-in done on day three of this week!!

Mind

When I was 28, I did my first real jumping jack. At 31, I lifted my first real weight.

After so many years of having zero self-esteem, I've spent these last years filling my bucket with self-confidence, and filling what was once soft, shapeless skin with sexy, shapely muscle. And sometimes, you know what, I'm gonna show it off. You know why? Because mama didn't just go to the store and buy that ass, and that ass is not gonna look the way it does now forever. Ain't nobody gonna tell me I can't show it off.

Have you got anything you want to show off? I say, if you got it, flaunt it. If you worked to achieve anything, a new job, a degree, whatever, I say be proud as fuck of that accomplishment. That doesn't mean you have to brag about it, but I don't see why we can't be openly happy about our achievements and in turn be openly celebratory about what others achieve.

I want you to carry these thoughts with you this week. Do the work and celebrate it, and at the same time applaud others who are brave enough to say too: *Yeah, I did that.* Let's bring each other up!

Muscle

Day One: Upper-Body Hybrid

Push-ups (can be done on knees): 4 × 10

Barbell flat chest presses: 4 × 30, 20, 15, 20

Dumbbell incline chest presses: 4 × 30, 20, 15, 20

Cable rows: 4 × 30, 20, 15, 20

Lat pull-downs (wide grip): 4 × 10–12

Lat V-bar pull-downs: 4 × 10–12

Biceps straight-bar curls: 4 × 20

Alternating biceps dumbbell curls: 4 × 10 (each arm)

Day Two: Cardio

Stairmaster: 30 minutes at steady speed (6.0)

Take 45–60 seconds between sets on the next exercises:

Drop squats (banded): 5 × 30

Banded diagonal-forward crab walks: 10 reps (each leg)

Mountain climbers: 3 × 30 seconds (take 30 seconds' rest between sets)

Day Three: Legs & Abs

Hip-ups (banded): 4 × 10 (with 1-second hold)

Squats (bodyweight): 5 × 10

Goblet squats: 4 × 10–12

Leg presses: 4 × 10–12

Quad extension machine: 4 × 20

Kneeling rope crunches: 4 × 20

Lying leg lifts: 3 × 30

Scissors: 3 × 30 (each leg)

Day Four: Upper-Body Hybrid

Pull-ups (band assisted): 4 × 10

Lat V-bar pull-downs: 4 × 10–12

Lat pull-downs (wide grip): 4 × 10–12

Biceps straight-bar curls: 4 × 15–20

Alternating biceps dumbbell curls: 4 × 10–12

Military presses: 4 × 15–20

Arnold presses: 4 × 10–12

Lateral raises: 4 × 15–20

Mouth: Follow-Up

Did you know that if your body believes it's starving, it will "correct" itself and send your metabolism into fat-preservation mode? This is what happens when you use long-term low-calorie eating as a way to lose weight. You might initially lose weight, but at some point—the point at which your body says, "WTF! This is an emergency situation and we've got to hold on to this fat for when the shit really hits the fan!!"—your weight loss will stall. Why in the hell would your body decide to preserve fat? Because fat is the richest source of energy (your body is smarter than you), and fat equals survival when food is scarce. Your body adapts and adjusts to treat what was once a calorie deficit as maintenance. This is why you Must. Keep. Eating. I know this is a bit of a mindfuck because we've all been convinced that starvation is the only way to body salvation, but this is not true. You've got to nourish yourself, not just once in a while, but every single day!

Week 8

Month

I notice sometimes when I work with people that they have this strange fear of eating carbs at night. Well, I want to put an end to that myth. Carbs at night don't necessarily translate into weight gain. In fact, some people really like it because it helps them sleep better and feel fuller.

Now, the quality of the carbs you eat means everything, so please don't go to bed eating Oreo cookies as your carb intake, even if you somehow manage to fit it into your macros, LOL. In this case, quality matters, and opting for the best quality will always maximize your results.

Day four of this week is your 10-day check-in day!! You know what to do. This means you'll be eating whatever caloric conclusion you come to, whether it's the same or 100 calories up or down, on the first day of the next rotation.

Mind

As your commitment to yourself deepens, I challenge you to start to say NO to things and feelings that just don't serve you anymore. When you say NO to people and things and even to yourself in the process of becoming a better you, you will begin to see, in how people react or respond, their true intentions.

If they understand and stay and help you in your endeavors, you will grow, and they will grow, and they will become part of your ever-evolving life, and vice versa.

If they (people, things, even your own feelings) can't handle your NOs, then they will slowly but surely disappear. It will feel strange at first, but this is actually not a bad thing—it just means, at this point, dividing paths are okay. This is true for anything: jobs, friends, relationships. The more you say NO to external things that may not be the best for you, the more you will open up your life to new and positive experiences—and the more empowered you will feel to do the things that create a better you. Saying no doesn't make you an asshole; it just means you're putting YOU first and the people, things, jobs, and feelings that care will stick around and watch you slay.

Muscle

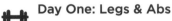 **Day One: Legs & Abs**

Lying leg lifts: 4 × 20

Scissors: 4 × 20 (each leg)

Mountain climbers: 3 × 30 seconds (take 30 seconds' rest between sets)

High knees: 3 × 20 seconds (each leg; take 30 seconds' rest between sets)

Dead lifts: 5 × 10

Dumbbell stiff-leg dead lifts: 4 × 10, 12

Leg presses (wide stance): 4 × 10, 12

Hamstring extension machine: 5 × 20

Adductor machine: 4 × 20

Day Two: Movement Hybrid

Stairmaster: 25 minutes at steady speed

Military presses: 4 × 10, 15

Plyo split lunges: 4 × 10 (each leg)

Drop squats (banded): 4 × 20

KB swings: 4 × 40 (find a weight that challenges you!)

Goblet squats: 4 × 20

Jump rope: 5 minutes

Day Three: Upper Body & Cardio

Seated V-bar cable rows: 4 × 15, 20

Lat pull-downs (wide grip): 4 × 12, 15

Bent-over dumbbell rows: 4 × 10 (together)

Biceps rope curls: 4 × 20

Biceps barbell curls: 4 × 12, 15

Alternating biceps dumbbell curls: 4 × 10

Bicycle sprints: 10 minutes (alternate 15 seconds' sprinting with 45 seconds at a normal pace for 10 minutes)

······························· *Mel's Tip* ·······························
Bike sprints are fucking hell, but they are effective, efficient, and great for delivering immediate gratification, which is what everyone wants, right?!

Day Four: Legs & Shoulders
Squats (bodyweight): 4 × 20

Squats (wide stance): 4 × 10

Leg presses: 4 × 10

Quad extension machine: 4 × 15, 20

Hamstring extension machine: 4 × 15, 20

Seated calf raises: 4 × 10, 15

Military presses: 4 × 20

Arnold presses: 4 × 10

Lateral raises: 4 × 15, 20

Mouth: Follow-Up

Roll call for macros: Carbs, protein, and fat—you all present? Check your diet and make sure! You need foods from each category to ensure that your body is getting what it needs to build that better body you want. If you're feeling a little bored, try to mix things up a little by paying attention to fiber. (Everyone knows fiber brings the F-U-N to any party.)

Fiber can help you feel full and keep your blood sugar in check—this will help prevent crazy-intense cravings for crappy carbs like chips and candy bars, and make sure your digestion doesn't stall after you've made some dietary adjustments. Just make sure to drink plenty of water along with any increase in fibrous foods!

Chapter Five

90°

Did you know that even if you aren't a natural-born badass, you can become one?

You've completed two months of The Turnaround—fuck, yes! Your opinion of yourself has changed: You feel confident and committed, and you're feeling a little bit addicted to the weekly changes your body is making. You still have no idea what's to come, but you now believe, and with this you've opened up a whole other can of whoop-ass on yourself. That's why this rotation is all about *dedication over motivation*. You'll see why.

MIND

Okay, so at this point you will be physically and mentally stronger, and it'll feel better than you thought. "Holy shit! I can't believe that two months have gone by," you'll say. Yeah, you hit a few speed bumps, but duh, it's the beginning of a whole new experience. If you didn't, I'd be worried and you wouldn't be reading this book, Supergirl (insert eyeroll emoji).

So far, you've done exactly what you were supposed to do, and you are exactly where you need to be. You're right on track, you finally (somewhat) got your shit together after so many attempts, and though you're not at your final destination, your weight has changed, you've built muscle, and your body is looking more like someone who actually gives a shit about themselves—it's smooth sailing from here, right? Not so fast. It's right about now that you're at risk of losing motivation because you have enough results to feel a temptation to slack off. You can get ahead of this temptation by knowing what's to come. Here's what you can expect:

A CONFRONTATION WITH YOUR PAST. Expect to have to decide between saying yes to your future self and your commitment or going back to your old habits. Say yes to your better future all day, every day. That bitch from your past can be tricky and tempting, though, saying things like, "Remember when we were wild and free, and you were just happy in your unhappiness?" Discontent can feel like a comfy old couch. But you've moved out, moved on, and that couch is sitting at Goodwill. Don't be the person who goes to the thrift store to buy back their own old stuff.

DISTRACTIONS EVERYWHERE. You will find yourself trying to come up with excuses not to do the work, and you'll discover that it feels like shit when you listen to those excuses. Sometimes, though, these excuses are a cry for a proper break on your day off. The reality is that your body has been going hard and it needs rest and play to make it grow and change, just as much as a plant needs sunshine to flourish. Be sure to be just as committed to your recovery time as you are your workout time, because your body (and brain) needs this desperately. Schedule rest and recovery as if it's part of your routine, and this will help you be more equipped to stay on track. I've also scheduled some solid rest time for you in this rotation—watch for it after Week 12's workouts.

AN UNEXPECTED DECREASE IN MOTIVATION. Believe it or not, this is not a bad thing, because it means you're entering pro status. You no longer need motivation to move forward; working out has become a habit and skipping days just doesn't feel okay anymore. Your dedication is now driving you forward. What does this mean? It means that there are still days when you wake up thinking, *No fucking way am I getting up today to work out.* (P.S. This is NORMAL. You're not a perfect little robot.) But you do it anyway, again and again. Because there's some crazy sort of deep-sea-level dedication that you've tapped into (I'm talking cellular shit that you didn't even know you had in you), and it's driving this ship now.

I've found that this is a good time to pause and ask yourself some questions. Of course, asking isn't worth shit unless you're ready to provide real, honest answers. Ask yourself these questions and, to protect against little lies or "creative truths" (i.e., rationalizing your bullshit), write down your answers in print. Yes, in print—go old school and bust out a pen and paper for this process. It's tougher to lie to yourself when you have to write it out *and* see the answers staring back at you in solid form. So, get your Bic out and be brave. Ask yourself:

- Have I been following the program to the best of my ability?

- Am I trying my hardest?

- Am I happy with my progress and results at this point?

- Are there things I wish I was doing or could be doing better?

If you've made mistakes, that's okay; that's what's supposed to happen when you try new stuff. Success comes from failure. But if you answered an honest "NO" to the question of whether or not you're trying your hardest, ask yourself, "Why not?" And then write down the excuse you have in your back pocket because you know you've been saving that shit for this very moment. Now, ask yourself, "Is this a valid excuse?" Or is it just that you've fallen onto your old, familiar, comfy couch? If it's the latter, get up off of that couch. It's nasty, dank, and dusty, and you're done with that shit!!

MOUTH

At this point, you have been working on consistency and found a set of meals that delivered results for you. You're in a groove, things don't take SOOO much work, and you kind of have your fave meals. Finally, you are cooking at least three-quarters of the stuff you buy instead of eating out of a takeout box three times a day, every damn day (and feeling lousy about the healthy, quality food you wasted). This shit is feeling like a lifestyle. Finally, damn it! Feels good, right?! Yes, it does! The more you do this, the easier it becomes, and pretty soon you'll be eating on point without even thinking about it.

In this rotation, you might find yourself flipping through the dessert pages in the recipe section and at least eyeing the pastries at the grocery store with a sense of having earned them. Your mind starts the chatter around justifying "little" treats and cheats. Your mind will tell you, *Have some more peanut butter—it's all good, you are doing great.* Yes, you're doing great, and some peanut butter can't take that away, but when you get to a good place, all the old habits that put you in a bad place will do their absolute best to bring you back there. In other words, just be careful when you start listening to that convincing little voice because it can get louder and more demanding once you give in even a little bit.

Personally, I fucking LOVE cheat snacks, treats, meals, whatever. You've probably learned over these last several weeks that it is almost impossible not to indulge—suddenly you probably feel like you're living on temptation island. Honestly, though, you should indulge sometimes. However, you have to earn the cheat. I personally have one cheat meal—not a cheat day—every 10 days. My go-to is having some nice dinner at a really good restaurant and finishing off with some dessert—I love cake. You can make the call for yourself on whether or not you want to incorporate this cheat meal every 10 days or so for yourself—only you can say how slippery the slope back to unhealthy eating is for you! (This cheat option only applies once you're in the 90-degree rotation—if you're peeking ahead here, you don't get cheats just yet!!)

Now, that doesn't mean you should go about having a cheat every day or "just a couple of drinks after work" whenever you have a tough day. These are all excuses—you need to put your goals first and EARN the cheat, earn the abs, and earn the physique you want.

It's time to get uncomfortable again! Learn to make some of the other recipes you haven't tried, switch the protein from one recipe and carbs from another.

The Imperfect Science of Meal Prep

You may have meal-prepped a few times and had to throw away some of the food, and that's normal. If you eat through four out of seven of your meal prep servings, you're good; only psychos get through 100% of their meal prep anyways. P.S., I'm not encouraging you to waste food—just trying to prevent you from beating yourself up about anything. As with everything else, you will get better at meal prep as you do it more!

MUSCLE

At this very moment, the one that happens right before you get started on the 90-degree rotation, you can expect to feel:

- More confident—you no longer feel like you look like a complete moron in the gym.

- A lot stronger—you can't even believe it: Your strength surprises you in everyday ways that you didn't anticipate.

- Like your mind-muscle connection is finally showing up (at least in some places). You'll notice this connection is stronger in your more developed muscles, which is normal. Your nerves and muscles work together to create engagement, so the bigger muscles are easier to communicate with—they're just a larger target for your brain to talk to!

- As though you now know what "The Pump" feels like; that is, the sensation when you feel your muscles actually working (that tightness and fatigue).

- Not as sore anymore because you're in better shape (soreness doesn't necessarily mean results).

As far as your weight goes, you've definitely lost some weight, but maybe not as much as you expected. What you notice, though, is that it doesn't matter because your body is looking and feeling tighter and some muscle definition is coming in.

You may start wondering at this point if you need special gloves, straps, wraps, shoes, belts, etc.—but I still stand by my position that you don't need any of that. It won't help you get results faster, and you may actually start to sneak in some bad form if you use aids this early in the process.

I guess if you want gloves so that you don't get calluses, that would be acceptable—but you really don't need anything. I personally love calluses because I feel like they're a telltale sign of hard work! But it's okay if they're not your thing.

THE TURNAROUND 90°: WEEKS 9–17 CALENDAR

It's time to lose fat and make some more muscle! This month is all about pushing the weight and honing your skills—you're getting ready to train at a higher level. Expect the results to start pouring in. Let's get the grind going!

Week 9

Mouth

How accurate have you been with tracking calories? By accurate I mean actually hitting your macros rather than purposely being "a little short" on carbs, for example. STOP. To change your body, you need to be serious and consistent. I know, because I did the same: People tend to be short on carbs and avoid eating their veggies in an effort to low-key eat less, because they still don't believe that you need to eat to lose weight. So, instead of being short, use the Nutrient-Rich Sides section of the recipes to complete your intake for the day since you can choose rice, eggplant, and even broccoli to complete what you need and be absolutely on point. Here's a sample of what I'd eat every day this week:

> Meal 1: Overnight Oats and Chia Bowl
> Meal 2: Whole Tandoori Roasted Chicken + Brown Rice + Asparagus
> Mela 3: Guacamole with Sweet Potato Chips + Chicken
> Meal 4: Mushroom Frittata + Baby Spinach

Mind

Here's the truth: YOU ARE AWAKE RIGHT NOW. Pinch yourself. You get to have this day, and you get to decide what you want to do with it. Quit your doubts, drop your demons off at daycare (if you haven't dumped them completely yet), and take a solid breath in of that precious air. Feel fucking grateful that you have the opportunity to be in a place where one of the "struggles" you have to overcome is whether or not you can get your shit in shape. Where I come from, this is called lucky as shit. YOU ARE AWAKE. And you can't go back to sleep without feeling regret or guilt, so just keep on going.

Muscle

Day One: Chest & Triceps

Perform 4 sets of each exercise:

Barbell flat chest presses: 8–12 reps

Dumbbell incline chest presses: 8–12 reps

Pec decks: 8–12 reps

Skull crushers (incline bench and E-Z bar): 8–12 reps

Triceps cable push-downs (straight bar): 20 reps

To be done after the 4 sets:

Sprints: 10 minutes on treadmill (alternate 30 seconds' sprinting with 30 seconds' walking, for a total of 10 minutes)

Day Two: Legs

Perform 4 sets of each exercise:

Quad extension machine: 20 reps

Squats (wide stance): 8–12 reps

Walking lunges (bodyweight): 12 reps (each leg)

Leg presses (narrow stance): 8–12 reps

Standing calf raises: 20 reps

Kick-backs (bodyweight): 5 × 30 (each leg)

Day Three: Back & Biceps

Perform 4 sets of each exercise:

Barbell rows (supinated grip): 8–12 reps (1-second hold in the back)

Lat pull-downs (wide grip): 8–12 reps

Seated V-bar cable rows: 8–12 reps (1-second hold in the back)

Reverse pec decks: 8–12 reps

Biceps straight-bar curls: 8–12 reps

Dumbbell incline biceps curls: 20 reps

Day Four: Legs

Perform 4 sets of each exercise:

Hamstring extension machine: 8–12 reps

Goblet squats: 8–12 reps

Leg presses (wide stance): 8–12 reps (fluid reps)

Hip thrusts (barbell, banded): 8–12 reps (1-second pause at the top)

Sumo dead lifts: 8–12 reps (1-second hold at the bottom)

Adductor machine: 20–30 reps

Kick-backs (bodyweight): 5 × 30 (each leg)

Day Five: Shoulders & Abs

Perform 4 sets of each exercise:

Seated shoulder presses: 8–12 reps

Military presses: 8–12 reps

Front raises: 20 reps

Face pulls: 20 reps

Kneeling rope crunches: 20–30 reps

Decline sit-ups: 12 reps (2–3 seconds on the way down)

To be done after the 4 sets:

Sprints: 10 minutes on treadmill (alternate 30 seconds' sprinting with 30 seconds' walking, for a total of 10 minutes)

Week 10

Mouth

How about I tell you what to eat? We are both eating the same this week, just adjust the quantities to your specific macros. You can find all these delicious dishes in the recipes section, of course:

Meal 1: Egg-Salad-Stuffed Celery

Meal 2: Ground Turkey Kofta + White Rice + Asparagus

Meal 3: Roasted Chicken with Peperonata + Cauliflower

Meal 4: Beef and Broccoli

On day three of this week it's time for your 10-day check-in. Check it. Change it, or not. Your results will tell you what to do.

Mind

 I know I've been talking to you (and YELLING AT YOU a little) over a lot of pages at this point and I just want to pause here and tell you something (something that I wish someone would say to me sometimes): You are going to make it.

Read that one more time. Yeah, that line right above this.

Whatever shit you have going on right now—and I'm not talking about whatever you have going on with The Turnaround, I'm talking about the hard stuff outside of here: the funky headspace, the tough relationships, the exhausting job, the asshole boss, the sick kid, the annoying parent, the money panic, the moral panic ("How bad did I just fuck up that friendship??"), the sibling rivalry that you thought you all would have grown out of by now, the "Shit, is life going to be like this every damn day?"—you know, all of that unavoidable life stuff, you are going to make it through it all. Not only that, but you are going to use whatever sort of mess you have in your own personal life as fuel for your commitment to yourself. Because when you think of all of *that*, doesn't a workout dedicated to your own betterment sound like a safe place of solace? Your time in the gym can be exactly that for you, if you learn to see it that way. I hope you've learned to cherish it. I know it's saved me a time or two, or two thousand.

Muscle

Day One: Chest & Triceps

Perform 4 sets of each exercise:

Barbell incline chest presses: 8–12 reps

Dumbbell flat chest presses: 8–12 reps

Pec decks: 8–12 reps

E-Z bar skull crushers on bench: 8–12 reps

Triceps cable push-downs (straight bar): 20 reps

To be done after the 4 sets:

Sprints: 10 minutes on treadmill (alternate 30 seconds' sprinting with 30 seconds' walking, for a total of 10 minutes)

Day Two: Legs

Perform 4 sets of each exercise:

Squats (wide stance): 8–12 reps

Quad extension machine: 20 reps

Walking lunges (bodyweight): 12 reps (each leg)

Leg presses (wide stance): 8–12 reps

Seated calf raises: 20 reps

Kick-backs (bodyweight): 30 reps (each leg)

Day Three: Back & Triceps

Perform 4 sets of each exercise:

Barbell rows (supinated grip): 8–12 reps (1-second hold in the back)

Lat pull-downs (supinated narrow grip): 8–12 reps

Seated V-bar cable rows: 8–12 reps (1-second hold in the back)

Reverse pec decks: 8–12 reps

Biceps straight-bar curls: 8–12 reps

Alternating biceps dumbbell curls: 20 reps (each arm)

Day Four: Legs

Perform 4 sets of each exercise:

Sumo dead lifts: 8–12 reps (1-second hold at the bottom)

Goblet squats: 8–12 reps

Hamstring extension machine: 8–12 reps

Leg presses (wide stance): 8–12 reps (fluid reps)

Hip thrusts (barbell, banded): 8–12 reps (1-second pause at the top)

Adductor machine: 20–30 reps

Crab walks (bodyweight): 10 reps (each leg)

Day Five: Shoulders & Abs

Perform 4 sets of each exercise:

Military presses: 8–12 reps

Seated shoulder presses: 8–12 reps

Lateral raises: 20 reps

Face pulls: 20 reps

Kneeling rope crunches: 20–30 reps

Decline sit-ups: 12 reps (2–3 seconds on the way down)

To be done after the 4 sets:

Sprints: 10 minutes on treadmill (alternate 30 seconds' sprinting with 30 seconds' walking, for a total of 10 minutes)

Week 11

Mouth

 On some days, an egg may save your life—or at least your job or your relationship. Just hear me out. Unaddressed hunger can make you do and say crazy things, *hangry* things. And you might have noticed that the hunger you experience when you're working your body as hard as you are is a different sort of beast, one that is a bit more demanding, urgent, and deep. That's where the humble egg comes in. It's a perfect little package of protein and nutrients all rolled into one. That's why you should always have eggs in your fridge. If you come home from work starving, cook up a couple eggs quickly before you make a decision to eat your kid's leftover mac and cheese or a whole bag of Doritos. Or if you're desperate for a snack somewhere, ask if they have hardboiled eggs (they're pretty popular these days—even 7-Eleven has been known to carry them).

Check it: Your 10-day check-in should happen on day six of this week!

Mind

Next time, someone says to you, "*Damn*, you look great," try saying, "Thank you. I've lost a lot of layers of bullshit over the last couple of months." (I mean, how awesome would it be to really say that to someone? If you do it, PLEASE hit me up on IG and tell me how it went down!!)

The truth is, you would not be lying; as you've worked to uncover your potential over the last several weeks, you have no doubt dropped some serious bullshit baggage. Even though this is a good thing, once these protective layers are removed, you can be left with a lot of exposed hope and optimism. And this can feel surprisingly scary—what if you actually get what you've always wanted? What happens then? Who are you when you can't hide behind a wall of excuses and disappointment? If you feel a little scared, you are going in the right direction—keep going, girl.

Muscle

 Day One: Chest & Triceps

Perform 4 sets of each exercise:

Push-ups: 10–15 reps

Barbell incline chest presses: 8–12 reps

Dumbbell incline chest presses: 8–12 reps

Triceps cable pull-downs (rope): 8–12 reps

Skull crushers (incline bench and E-Z bar): 8–12 reps

Triceps cable push-downs (straight bar): 20 reps

To be done after the 4 sets:

Sprints: 10 minutes on treadmill (alternate 30 seconds' sprinting with 30 seconds' walking, for a total of 10 minutes)

Day Two: Legs

Perform 4 sets of each exercise:

Quad extension machine: 20 reps

Squats (wide stance): 8–12 reps

Walking lunges with dumbbells: 12 reps (each leg)

Leg presses (narrow stance): 8–12 reps

Standing calf raises: 20 reps

Kick-backs (bodyweight): 30 reps (each leg)

Day Three: Back & Biceps

Perform 4 sets of each exercise:

Barbell rows (supinated grip): 8–12 reps (1-second hold in the back)

Lat pull-downs (wide grip): 8–12 reps

Seated V-bar cable rows: 8–12 reps (1-second hold in the back)

Reverse pec decks: 8–12 reps

Biceps straight-bar curls: 8–12 reps
Dumbbell incline biceps curls: 20 reps

Day Four: Legs
Perform 4 sets of each exercise:
Hamstring extension machine: 8–12 reps
Goblet squats: 8–12 reps
Leg presses (wide stance): 8–12 reps (fluid reps)
Hip thrusts (barbell, banded): 8–12 reps (1-second pause at the top)
Sumo dead lifts: 8–12 reps (1-second hold at the bottom)
Adductor machine: 20–30 reps
Hip-ups (banded): 20 reps

Day Five: Shoulders & Abs
Perform 4 sets of each exercise:
Seated shoulder presses: 8–12 reps
Military presses: 8–12 reps
Front raises: 20 reps
Face pulls: 20 reps
Kneeling rope crunches: 20–30 reps
Decline sit-ups: 12 reps (2–3 seconds on the way down)

To be done after the 4 sets:
Sprints: 10 minutes on treadmill (alternate 30 seconds' sprinting with 30 seconds' walking, for a total of 10 minutes)

Week 12

Mouth

Shit has been getting serious in the gym for a while now, and you are probably feeling like you're getting stronger and making progress literally every day. Despite the popular belief that you need a bunch of protein to make pretty muscles, the truth is that carbs play a huge role in the recovery process. I recommend getting a solid meal with tons of carbs after your workout so that you can get that recovery process jump-started. Here's my post-workout go-to meal due to its ease of preparation, packability, and ability to add or subtract certain macros:

Beef and Broccoli + Sweet Potatoes

Mind

 I have a confession to make: I cry all the time. For real. I don't want you to be under the false impression that because I've got abs and biceps and back muscles, and I can smile and be goofy in the gym, I'm living some kind of perfect life. Far from it. I still struggle with self-confidence, self-doubt, and uncertainty all the time. What's different now, though, is that these thoughts and feelings used to form a sort of all-consuming sea around me—I would feel myself swimming in that shit all day long. No matter how hard I tried, I couldn't get away from the doubts and insecurities. But making a dedication to my goals helped me step out of that sea and up onto the shore. Now, that shit rises up like the tide and nips at my feet and legs, and threatens to pull me in, but my commitment and purpose, and the fact that I have proved to myself that I can be consistent, reliable, and strong, help me resist against the pull of that current. (The only way I'm ever going back into that sea is when I can sail back into that shit on a motherfuckin' yacht—a girl can dream.)

My point is that sometimes it's okay to not be okay. You're a work in progress, just like me, just like everyone. No one has it all figured out. If they tell you they do, they're full of shit. So, you keep working your way out of whatever sea you might be stuck in—the work will get you out.

Muscle

Day One: Chest & Triceps
Perform 4 sets of each exercise:
Pull-ups (band assisted): 10 reps
Barbell incline chest presses: 8–12 reps
Dumbbell flat chest presses: 8–12 reps
Push-ups: 8–12 reps
E-Z bar skull crushers on bench: 8–12 reps
Triceps cable push-downs (straight bar): 20 reps

To be done after the 4 sets:

Sprints: 10 minutes on treadmill (alternate 30 seconds' sprinting with 30 seconds' walking, for a total of 10 minutes)

Day Two: Legs

Perform 4 sets of each exercise:

Drop squats (banded): 20 reps

Squats (wide stance): 8–12 reps

Quad extension machine: 20 reps

Walking lunges with dumbbells: 12 reps (each leg)

Leg presses (wide stance): 8–12 reps

Seated calf raises: 20 reps

Kick-backs (bodyweight): 30 reps (each leg)

Day Three: Back & Triceps

Perform 4 sets of each exercise:

Lateral jumping jacks: 30 reps

Barbell rows (supinated grip): 8–12 reps (1-second hold in the back)

Lat pull-downs (supinated narrow grip): 8–12 reps

Seated V-bar cable rows: 8–12 reps (1-second hold in the back)

Reverse pec decks: 8–12 reps

Triceps cable push-downs (straight bar): 8–12 reps

Alternating biceps dumbbell curls: 20 reps (each arm)

Day Four: Legs

Perform 4 sets of each exercise:

Kick-backs (bodyweight): 30 reps (each leg)

Sumo dead lifts: 8–12 reps (1-second hold at the bottom)

Goblet squats: 8–12 reps

Hamstring extension machine: 8–12 reps

Leg presses (wide stance): 8–12 reps (fluid reps)

Hip thrusts (barbell, banded): 8–12 reps (1-second pause at the top)

Adductor machine: 20–30 reps

Crab walks (bodyweight): 10 reps (each leg)

Day Five: Shoulders & Abs

Perform 4 sets of each exercise:

Jumping jacks: 50 reps

Lateral jumping jacks: 50 reps

Military presses: 8–12 reps

Seated shoulder presses: 8–12 reps

Lateral raises: 20 reps

Face pulls: 20 reps

Kneeling rope crunches: 20–30 reps

Decline sit-ups: 12 reps (2–3 seconds incline bench on the way down)

To be done after the 4 sets:

Sprints: 10 minutes on treadmill (alternate 30 seconds' sprinting with 30 seconds' walking, for a total of 10 minutes)

Week 13: Free Week

TAKE ONE WEEK OFF!!

DO NOT FREAK OUT—I haven't lost my mind! I know you're making tons of progress and you're in a super groove. So, why take a break now? You've completed several weeks of training, which has allowed you to create some killer results and your body is moving well. But this is the point where your body starts to accumulate wear and tear from usage (nothing to do with having good or bad form while training). Just like pro athletes or high-performance cars and bikes, your body needs a little reset in order to move on to the next level.

Now, I don't want you to sit on the couch for a week. I want you to walk, do yoga, keep getting massages, and do activities you enjoy. You also want to continue eating well and stay on track with your 10-day check-in, which will take place on the second day of your free week.

DO NOT skip the recovery week! You need to be fresh for what's coming. And trust me, you will discover how much you need these breaks! I recommend a week off roughly every 8–12 weeks for longevity and mental health.

 Get your 10-day check-in done on day two of this week!!

Week 14: Bringing It All Together

I hope that you took the suggested week off, because shit is about to get real! These next four weeks are all about taking your body and training to the next level. Be sure to eat accordingly (that is, according to the results you want to see—if you want to work your ass off in the gym and not see it pay off as much as it could, go ahead and eat like crap; ain't nobody stopping you). BUT if you want to see the best possible outcome, results-wise, you know how you should be eating.

Mouth

 How are you sleeping? If you're physically tired, as opposed to mentally tired, at the end of the day and falling asleep like a baby, you're very lucky and I'm very happy. If you are struggling a bit or if you're waking up feeling a little beat up, maybe more than normal, then I recommend you have more carbs during your last meal right before bed. Yup, you heard correctly! Real food carbs will cause an insulin spike and help you fall asleep, then you will be digesting them and repairing your muscle energy reserves while you sleep, which will translate to better mornings. BOOM!

Here are some of my favorite carbs to enjoy at dinner:

White rice
Sweet potatoes
Eggplant

Of the three, eggplant is probably my favorite because it's delicious and it also allows me to eat a ton of it due to its low-carb macros. Notice how I actually eat carbs at dinner!

 On day five of this week, it's time for your 10-day check-in.

Mind

This is what every journey looks like:

Confusion
Excitement
Attempt

Failure
More failure
Success
YOU'RE ON THE RIGHT PATH!!

Muscle

 Day One: Legs
Squats (bodyweight): 80 reps
Squats (wide stance): 5 × 10 (3 seconds on the way down, 1-second hold at the bottom, drive up with power or 3,1,0 tempo)

Tempo Tiempo

In this week's workouts, you'll see I introduced something called "*tempo*," which is a more specific time assignment to the different phases of your movements. I like incorporating tempo because it's a reminder that moving a weight up and down, or back and forth, is NOT lifting weights; it takes focused control to engage your nerves and muscles fully and to maximize growth and flexibility.

Generally, stretching/lengthening movements (think coming down to a squat as stretching your quad muscles) need to happen with steady movement plus control (i.e., it should take 1–2 seconds), while coming back up (squeezing/shortening quad muscles) happens a little faster with more engagement (about 1 second or less). The official term for stretch movement is "eccentric" and for the squeeze part it's "concentric." So, you may hear something like "1-second pause on the eccentric," which means to pause at the bottom of the squat for 1 second.

When you see "tempo" in The Turnaround workouts, this simply means that I want you to be a little more strategic about the seconds you spend on each rep. For example, a 3,1,0 tempo with a squat will mean taking three seconds on the way down, holding and squeezing for one second, and then driving up with power. In some cases, tempo times will appear in shorthand as three numbers after the prescribed sets and reps—so "4 × 10, 2,0,0" will mean four sets of 10 reps done at 2,0,0 tempo. Tempo times will vary depending on the exercise and the rest of the movements you're doing within a specific workout.

While you won't see a tempo note on every exercise, you can apply the intention, which is to avoid jittery, out-of-control, wobbly, or otherwise poor movement patterns, to just about any physical moves you make.

Single-leg lying hamstring extensions: 4 × 10 (3,1,0 tempo)
Single-leg quad extensions: 4 × 10 (3,1,0 tempo)
Walking lunges with dumbbells: 4 × 12–15 (each leg, 2 seconds on the way down)
Hip-ups (banded): 4 × 12–15 (1-second pause at the top)
Kick-backs (bodyweight): 4 × 50 (each leg)

Day Two: Chest & Biceps & Abs
Push-ups: 4 × 10
Dumbbell flat chest presses: 5 × 10 (2,0,0 tempo)
Cable chest flies: 4 × 10 (1-second hold)
Biceps barbell curls: 4 × 10
Biceps straight-bar curls: 4 × 10
Alternating biceps dumbbell curls: 4 × 12
Kneeling rope crunches: 5 × 20
Incline leg lifts: 4 × 20
Stairmaster: 15 minutes (6.0)

Day Three: Legs
Squat-lunge-squat-lunges: 3 × 10
Dead lifts: 4 × 10 (3,1,0 tempo)
Hip thrusts (barbell, banded): 4 × 10 (1-second pause at the top)
Sumo squats (Smith machine): 4 × 10 (fluid reps)
Good mornings: 4 × 10
Standing calf raises: 5 × 10 (1-second hold at the top)
Kick-backs (bodyweight): 4 × 50 (each leg)

Day Four: Back & Triceps & Shoulders
Lateral jumping jacks: 100 reps
Pull-ups (band assisted): 4 × 10 (controlled movement on the way down)
Bent-over Smith machine rows (supinated grip): 4 × 10
Banded straight-arm pull-downs: 4 × 12–15
Assisted dips: 4 × 12–15
Face pulls: 4 × 12–15

Front raises and lateral raises: 4 × 10+10
Stairmaster: 15 minutes (6.0)

Day Five: Legs
Drop squats (banded): 2 × 20
Hip thrusts (barbell, banded): 4 × 10 (1-second pause at the top)
Sumo dead lifts: 5 × 10 (3,1,0 tempo)
Walking lunges with dumbbells: 4 × 10 (each leg, 2 seconds on the way down)
Dumbbell stiff-leg dead lifts: 4 × 10 (3,1,0 tempo)
Banded step-outs: 4 × 10 (each leg)
Kick-backs (bodyweight): 5 × 30 (each leg)

Week 15

Mouth

Water intake check—do you know how much water you're drinking each day? You should. Drinking water seems like such a basic thing, yet most people can't keep up the 100+ ounces of water per day (per day, as in every day, not 100 ounces one day and then 10 ounces the next) that I recommend. If you have been killing the water game and easily going through at least a gallon per day, keep it up! If you haven't, then it's time we go back to the basics and start lugging that giant water bottle around again—think about it as an arm workout rather than something you have to carry around. BTW, I always had a little acne here and there until I started drinking water like this: Hydration—and the food you're eating now—does wonders for your skin!

Mind

YO! I've got something to tell you, and it's sort of like a game of telephone except after I tell you, you tell yourself and not someone else, and you don't mess up the words—so it's not really like telephone at all. In fact it's way more important than that, so I'll get serious for a sec. Here's what I want you to know:

- You are strong.
- You are smart.
- You are beautiful.

- You can do anything you want.
- You are in control.

You are all of those things. Don't forget it. And don't ever let anyone ever tell you otherwise.

Muscle

Day One: Legs
Crab walks (bodyweight): 3 × 10 (each leg)
Squats (wide stance): 4 × 12–15 (3,1,0 tempo)
Single-leg lying hamstring extensions: 4 × 12–15 (3,1,0 tempo)
Single-leg quad extensions: 4 × 12 (3,1,0 tempo)
Dumbbell static lunges: 4 × 12 (each leg, 2 seconds on the way down)
Hip thrusts (barbell, banded): 4 × 12–15 (1-second pause at the top)
Kick-backs (bodyweight): 5 × 30 (each leg)

Day Two: Chest & Biceps & Abs
Jumping jacks: 100 reps
Dumbbell incline chest presses: 4 × 12 (2,0,0 tempo)
Cable chest flies: 4 × 15–20
Biceps barbell curls: 4 × 12–15
Biceps straight-bar curls: 4 × 12–15
Dumbbell incline biceps curls: 4 × 10
Kneeling rope crunches: 5 × 20
Incline leg lifts: 4 × 20
Stairmaster: 15 minutes (6.0)

Day Three: Legs
Banded diagonal-forward crab walks: 3 × 10 (each leg)
Dead lifts: 4 × 12–15 (3,1,0 tempo)
Hip thrusts (barbell, banded): 4 × 12–15 (1-second pause at the top)
Goblet squats: 4 × 12–15 (fluid reps)
Good mornings: 4 × 12–15

Seated calf raises: 4 × 12–15 (1-second hold at the top)
Kick-backs (bodyweight): 4 × 50 (each leg)

Day Four: Back & Triceps & Shoulders
Push-ups: 3 × 10
Bent-over dumbbell rows: 4 × 12–15
Pull-ups (band assisted): 4 × 12–15 (controlled movement on the way down)
Banded straight-arm pull-downs: 4 × 20
Assisted dips: 4 × 12–15
Face pulls: 4 × 20
Front raises and lateral raises: 4 × 10+10
Stairmaster: 15 minutes (6.0)

Day Five: Legs
Crab walks (bodyweight): 2 × 15 (each leg)
Sumo dead lifts: 5 × 12 (3,1,0 tempo)
Hip thrusts (barbell, banded): 4 × 12 (1-second pause at the bottom)
Dumbbell static lunges: 4 × 12 (each leg, 2 seconds on the way down)
Dumbbell stiff-leg dead lifts: 4 × 12–15 (3,1,0 tempo)
Banded step-outs: 4 × 15–20 (each leg)
Kick-backs (bodyweight): 5 × 30 (each leg)

Week 16

Mouth

Avoid food knockoffs as often as possible. By now, you probably got "smart" and figured you can buy canned or boxed versions of the ingredients you need to create my recipes, or you can simply manipulate these foods to fit your macros. And while you can make canned beans, boxed rice, and "fiber crisps" fit into your macros, I need to remind you that these are knockoff versions of unprocessed food. The closer the food item is to its natural/raw state, the easier it will be for your body to digest and turn it into the pretty, strong, flexible muscles you're looking to make. In addition, you will literally be healthier, inside and out, by going for the real deal as much as possible.

Get your 10-day check-in done on day one of this week!!

Mind

 Tips on how to be the fucking best:

1. Do not care what people think.

2. Scream, cry, curse.

3. Love yourself like it's your job.

4. Be kind to everyone you meet. (Except for that bro who stole your squat rack—he gets a whole lotta attitude. And those people who put a milk carton with just a dribble back in the fridge—WTF. And for dudes who leave the toilet seat up or the ones who put the empty bag of cereal back in the box or the last person who uses all the toilet paper and doesn't replace the roll, arrgggggg! You can unload on them. But be nice to everyone else.)

5. And once more, for those of you in the back: Don't care what people think! No one else pays your bills (or if they do, give 'em my number), squat your squats, get your butt up outta bed each day. Just do you and forget about the rest.

Muscle

 Same as Week 14 (pages 110–112)

Week 17

Mouth

By now you're extremely proficient at the tracking and nutrition game, so let me tell you what we'll be eating this week (as usual, modify portions according to your macros):

Meal 1: Shakshuka + Sweet Potatoes + Baby Spinach
Meal 2: Brown Rice Poke Bowl + Asparagus
Meal 3: Salmon with Broccolini + Eggplant
Meal 4: Bibimbap + Brussels Sprouts

Get your 10-day check-in done on day four of this week!!

Mind

 People are constantly looking for something they can call out as contradiction:

Oh, you the boss lady?
You can't cry when something pisses you off.

You're a stay-at-home mom?
You better have dinner on the table for your man/woman when they come home.

You a beast in the gym?
You must want to be a dude or something?

Muscle

 Same as Week 15 (pages 113–114)

Chapter Six

180°

The final rotation is all about MASTERING MANIFESTATION. With four months in, you've stepped out of the hand-holding zone—you are confident and capable and know your way around a gym. You now feel that you have all the tools; it's just a matter of determining for certain what you want to make of yourself. It is up to you to decide.

A curious thing happens at this point in The Turnaround—you are hungry for more, and you want to find out how much stronger you can get. You think and breathe desire for continued progress. Yet your body is not changing as fast as it was, or it might not even seem like it's changing at all. You experience a bit of a conflict—you think, "I know everything I need to know, but why do I now feel confused?" It's a tricky time, and I'm here to guide you all the way through it! I've been there, girl, many times before.

The beautiful thing is you now are so in sync with your body, so connected, that you know how to push it, know how to feed it, know how to help it recover. But you're at a beginning of sorts, a different next-level beginning than the one that came before. At this beginning, you have the freedom that knowledge brings and an awareness of who you are and who you want to be that will help you hone those goals until they are razor sharp.

MIND

 If you've made it here, your commitment to yourself and something big is legit, even legendary. Despite all the bumps, dips, sharp turns, and brick walls you no doubt ran into along the way, YOU MADE IT—and that is seriously awesome. (You can't see me right now, but I'm doing a little celebration dancey-dance in your honor.)

It doesn't matter what lingering doubts you have about yourself or how far you still think you have to go—you have changed your life in some amazing ways. I mean, you've probably proved to yourself that you can cook healthy foods that are lick-the-plate good, you can lift some heavy-ass metal in the morning and put your heels on in the evening and rock the club. You can feel sorer than you ever thought possible and kind of *like* it, so much that you've wanted to make sure to work out hard enough to feel it again. Who are you?!

But, enough praise. You've done good. But you still got work to do!

The work in the final weeks of The Turnaround is real and it's rough and you are ready for it; you've trained for this moment. I'm raising the game now because I know you can rise up to meet me at the top. You are not a beginner anymore. You are, however, in a way, back at square one. In this space, the changes will be smaller but more detailed, so be prepared. I want you to think of this rotation a little bit like you already bought your dream wedding dress and now you're tailoring it to fit just right.

MOUTH

At this point, you know so much more about food than you ever even wanted to know. And there are still some other food-related experiences you're going to have in the upcoming rotation:

GROCERY SHOPPING: Before, hitting the grocery store was something you did to simply prevent your fridge from being depressingly empty—I mean, let's face it: There are few things more depressing than opening a fridge and finding just a bottle of water and some old butter. Now, you *love* going to the supermarket and buying the food you like to cook; you're fantasizing about my recipes and bringing your own "secret twist" to some of them. Best of all, all this cooking instead of buying restaurant food means you're now eating higher-quality ingredients. Well done!

MEAL PREPPING: You make dinner and have leftovers for lunch the next day at work. You can make an amazing breakfast in under 20 minutes. Yup, you're no longer trying to meal prep for the entire week because you don't need to—you know already how to make food and utilize it throughout the week; it's just how you roll. Yo! You know what this means, don't you? You've got yourself a lifestyle choice! Keep it up.

RESULTS: You understand the relationship between nutrition and results, and this goes beyond calories. You are able to do something only a select group of the population can do: look at a food and establish its realistic nutritional value; determine if it's something you want (or if what you want is the better version of whatever it is); make an experience-based decision about what to eat and how this will or will not translate into results and performance that you actually want. I think this is a super cool, underrated life skill—you know how to power your own awesome life machine. Not many people can say that.

As you continue through this final rotation in The Turnaround, stay open to even more learning about eating and your relationship to food. It may be that your goal, training, and nutrition are all perfectly aligned at this point, but that wasn't the case for me when I started. The goal you defined in the beginning may not have been the healthiest thing for you. You might have discovered this to be the case, or you might still be in denial about this truth. And that's okay. Every day, every meal is an opportunity to accept what is the healthiest and best nutritional approach and look for your body. Just remember that you are in control of the choices you make, and you can make the right one. It may not be easy, even after so many weeks of putting in the work, but you are getting to know yourself and your needs, your *real* needs—your actions will catch up to meet those when the time is right.

MUSCLE

You are about to begin your 18th week on The Turnaround, and this means you have no doubt that I'm all about helping you build beautiful, bomb-ass muscle through the strategic use of weights and specific, wheels-on-fire (read: painful) spurts of cardio. Over the final weeks of the program, you're going to continue on in the same way with one important addition: It's time to mix it up! By mixing it up, I mean introducing some different types of movement. If you've been paying attention to your body, you can probably tell that it's been craving a little something different these days. You better give that girl what she wants, or else . . .

The truth is, I'm always surprised by how few people ask me about what else I do (or what else I tell my clients to do) other than lift weights. Yet these "other" things can be just as important as time spent in the gym because they're done for longevity, mobility, and recovery. The goal of introducing some additional types of activities is to work on your body's ability to move, and hopefully help it move better for longer. When you make some time to focus on mobilizing your joints and ligaments, and vary the way you fire up your muscles, you also help ensure that you get the most out of your training down the road.

In this rotation's weekly calendar, you'll see that a handful of "Active Recovery" days have been included. There are a few options for you to choose from, such as hot yoga and walking, so take your pick and enjoy. Keep in mind that these aren't meant to be free days. Steer your mind toward *why* you're doing this activity—maybe you're taking a yoga class for the breath work or walking to get centered or to improve your circulation after sitting at your damn desk all day. You can also try any other kind of activity you want that will challenge your body and brain in new ways. The goal is simply to gain something from whatever it is you choose.

THE TURNAROUND 180°: WEEKS 18–26 CALENDAR

It's time to chisel and define!

Week 18 (Heavy)

Mouth

You are now training at a level 400% higher than when we began. You should be eating without stress because you've realized that meal timing and avoiding carbs at night, etc., are mostly just BS—when you're putting in the work, you are rewarded with room for breaking these and other so-called rules of dieting! The only *real* rule is that you need to listen to your body: If you're hungry, eat! When I'm super hungry after training, I eat my Overnight Oats and Chia Bowl (page 184), and when I'm hungry *again* 1 or 2 hours later, I eat my Mushroom Frittata (page 180).

 Get your 10-day check-in done on day seven of this week!!

Mind

You are never too good for failure. The most impressive people I know are not afraid to keep challenging themselves, regardless of the risk of failure involved; they are willing to take a chance because it might mean growth and expansion, and it will certainly mean experience. The problem is when you get good or really good at something, it can start to feel hard to try new stuff because you develop this feeling that you have more to lose by trying something new. The potential for embarrassment seems that much greater.

I used to hate the thought of failure so much that if it seemed I was going to mess up at something, I would start to shake my head, like, "Oh, nuh-uh, no way this shit is going to make a fool of me." But eventually I realized that the most golden opportunities for growth are found when you go all in on trying new things.

I remember one new experience that I had, which was the first time that I had to accept an award—I won Create & Cultivate's Leading Figure in the Health and Wellness Space for 2018 award—and talk in front of hundreds of people, some of whom were also being awarded and saying cool AF things (by the way, #nopressure ugh) about things outside lifting weights and sweating. Well, I didn't know WTF to say other than the usual "Thank you." I had come to the awards show with my daughter, and I wanted her to be proud of her momma and bask in the moment—I wanted her to hear me say cool things that were memorable.

What did I do when I was finally standing there on stage, after stressing for days about what I was going to say? I turned my mind off, took a deep breath, and said what was in my heart while accepting the possibility that it may suck. Turns out it didn't suck at all; I said some clever things about the power of the mind and felt pretty damn inspired myself. My daughter may not remember this when she's older, but I will!

Anyways, sometimes you've gotta risk looking like a fool to learn about yourself and to grow. In my experience, people are too hard on themselves and things usually work out for the best if you do you and act from the heart.

So, I still freak out a little when I feel like a beginner again at anything. But I no longer shake my head; I grit my teeth and jump in, protected by the belief in myself and supported by my ability to always be the best at trying. I challenge you to get good at trying, too. In this sport, it's effort that counts. Success is one failure away, so get excited every time you "fail" because you're just that much closer to SUCCESS!

Muscle

Day One: Legs

Squat-lunge-squat-lunges: 3 × 10

Squats (bodyweight): 5 × 8–10

Bulgarian split squats: 4 × 10 (each leg)

Sumo squats (Smith machine): 4 × 10

Standing calf raises: 4 × 12–15

Drop squats (banded): 4 × 20

Bicycle sprints: 10 minutes (alternate 15 seconds' sprinting with 45 seconds at a normal pace for 10 minutes)

Day Two: Chest & Biceps

Push-ups: 4 × 10

Barbell incline chest presses: 5 × 8–10

Incline Smith machine presses: 3 × 10

Chest dips (assisted): 3 × 10

Biceps straight-bar curls: 4 × 20

Barbell preacher curls: 5 × 8–10

Alternating biceps dumbbell curls: 4 × 10

Day Three: Back & Triceps

Reverse pull-ups: 3 × 10

T-bar rows: 5 × 8–10

Bent-over rear delt barbell rows: 4 × 10

Reverse pec decks: 4 × 10

Triceps cable push-downs (straight bar): 3 × 20

Lying Smith machine triceps presses: 5 × 8–10

Seated triceps pull-overs: 4 × 10

Stairmaster: 10 minutes + 4 × 30 kick-backs (each leg)

Put this on a *giant* Post-it where you can see it every day: Don't get overconfident, because you're just one bad week away from deciding to go back the other way. Just. Keep. Going. I'm taking you so far forward that eventually there will be no going back.

Day Four: Legs

Walking lunges (bodyweight): 100 reps

Sumo squats: 4 × 8–10

Sumo dead lifts: 4 × 8–10

Hip thrusts (barbell, banded): 4 × 8–10 (1-second pause at the top)

Adductor machine: 4 × 20

Seated calf raises: 4 × 12–15

Day Five: Shoulders & Abs

Smith machine flat chest presses: 5 × 8–10

Standing dumbbell shoulder presses: 4 × 10

Single-arm dumbbell presses: 4 × 10 (each arm)

Hanging leg lifts: 4 × 15–20

Kneeling rope crunches: 4 × 20

Plank holds: 4 × 1 minute

Bicycle sprints: 10 minutes (alternate 15 seconds' sprinting with 45 seconds at a normal pace for 10 minutes)

Week 19 (Light-ish)

Mouth

Remember when you were a kid and the TV commercials all said that breakfast was the most important meal of the day, like so important that it's amazing you're alive if you don't eat breakfast? Yeah, made sense, sure, except that they were telling you to have cereal (highly processed sugar), some bacon (highly processed meat), and drink OJ for vitamin C (highly processed sugar). Guess what? If you want to train in the morning and go about your life, then eat later, around 10 a.m.—you will survive! You have learned by now that your body cares about nutrition over time, so don't stress about perfectly timing your meals or having "breakfast" food for breakfast.

Mind

As you've been strengthening your body over the past four months, you've also been strengthening your mind, whether you know it or not. And just as your physical muscles can now manage more weight, so too can those mental muscles of yours. Seriously, they are powerful as shit and capable of pushing you through even the toughest challenges. I want you to remember this when you find yourself unexpectedly entertaining those pesky doubt gremlins that enter your mind with the sole purpose of fucking things up. You know how to get rid of these guys? You ignore them, and you override those little punks with a focus on the present.

Doubts and insecurities feed off of attention, and it only makes them grow louder and stronger. But when you say "Hey!" and then move on, you debilitate their destructive ways. Test your brain next time they try you. Don't say to yourself, "NO, NO, NO, NO, the gremlins are fucking me over again. I'm such an idiot!"—trust me, that does not work. I've tried it a thousand times. Instead, learn to catch yourself when these thoughts show up as if you're a viewer of the thoughts. When the self-doubt and insecurities start creeping up, learn the pattern and at that moment say, "Oh, I'm starting to think about not being good enough and doubting myself. Okay, I see it. Well, that doesn't help. Let me focus on RIGHT NOW." And then look at your now. "Yup, I'm drinking my morning coffee and I love it, this is me time. Let me go and water my plants while I drink it."

Notice how I'm not telling you to yell at yourself for having those thoughts; instead I'm suggesting that you recognize them and simply shift your focus to the present and back to the things that add to your life. This will take practice, the same kind of practice that it's taken lifting weights all these weeks!!

Muscle

Day One: Legs
Lunges, alternating (bodyweight): 100 reps
Squats (bodyweight): 7 × 10 (fluid reps)
Quad extension machine: 4 × 20
Stationary forward-leaning lunges with dumbbells: 4 × 10 (each leg)

Banded diagonal-forward crab walks: 4 × 20
Standing calf raises: 4 × 10 (1-second hold at the top)
Stairmaster: 10 minutes + 4 × 30 kick-backs (each leg)

Day Two: Chest & Biceps
Push-ups: 3 × 10
Cable chest flies: 4 × 20
Smith machine flat chest presses: 4 × 10–12
Pec decks: 4 × 20
Barbell drag curls: 4 × 12–15
Alternating biceps dumbbell curls: 4 × 12 (each arm)
Shoulder taps (in plank position): 4 × 20 (tapping both shoulders is 1 rep)

······································· *Mel's Tip* ·······································
Train hard. Be intense. Have fun. Repeat.

Day Three: Legs & Shoulders
Sumo squats (Smith machine): 4 × 20
Banded hamstring curls: 4 × 20
Hip thrusts (bodyweight, banded): 4 × 12–15
Leg presses (wide stance): 4 × 12–15 (fluid reps)
Front raises: 4 × 12–15
Lateral raises: 4 × 12–15
Bicycle sprints: 10 minutes (alternate 15 seconds' sprinting with 45 seconds at a normal
    pace for 10 minutes)

Day Four: Back & Triceps
Pull-ups (band assisted): 4 × 10
Lat pull-downs (supinated narrow grip): 4 × 12–15
Single-arm dumbbell rows: 4 × 10 (each arm)
Bent-over rear delt barbell rows: 4 × 12–15
Standing rope triceps pull-overs: 5 × 20
Dips (bodyweight): 4 × 20

Day Five: Legs & Abs

Goblet squats: 3 × 20

Smith machine front squats: 4 × 12–15

Hip thrusts (barbell, banded): 4 × 12–15

Leg presses (wide stance and narrow stance): 4 × 10+10

Adductor machine: 4 × 20

Banded hamstring curls: 4 × 20

Lying leg lifts: 4 × 30

Stairmaster: 10 minutes + 4 × 30 kick-backs each leg

Week 20 (Heavy)

Mouth

Do you do the same activities during the workweek that you do on the weekends when you have more time? Yeah, I didn't think so. You probably feel a bit more structured and scheduled during the week and a little looser and fun on the weekends. I want you to apply this same separation to your eating habits. I want you to learn to enjoy the fruits of your hard work and freeing up how and what you eat should be part of this enjoyment. To get the fun into your food, be sure to check out my lunch/dinner recipes and let your palette do the rest. Gettin' fit and healthy shouldn't always feel like a chore.

 Get your 10-day check-in done on day three of this week!!

Mind

Watch out for that new comfort zone that you're settling into right about now. Sure, it's different from the one from before, and yeah, you probably *look* different—but inside you're still the same ol' human being. And us human beings seek comfort by nature. (Seriously, how quickly after you walk into a room do you start looking for somewhere to sit? Unless it's a mall, in which case you can walk for miles without food or water to find the right heels for that dress, riiiiiight?)

The truth is, we all want to feel safe and protected. Yet progress doesn't usually come out of safe places because progress and growth require pushing yourself, and that is uncomfortable. Seriously, that shit can hurt, physically and even more so emotionally. You're not a rookie anymore, so I know that you know all this already, but I'm just here right now to flash a little imaginary road sign at you: Caution: (New) Comfort Zone Ahead. Don't just speed right by; be sure to check in and ask yourself, *Am I too comfortable for progress to keep happening?* Keep grinding.

Muscle

Same as Week 18 (pages 122–123)

Week 21 (Light-ish)

Mouth

At this point in The Turnaround, most people have created enough results and experience that they start doing things a little lazy. You may find yourself skipping the micronutrients part of your meals, you know the baby spinach, arugula, broccoli, etc. DON'T. Although you may be hitting your macros, not entering the micros can have unwanted effects that can escalate fairly quickly. For example, if I skip my micros for a couple of days, all of a sudden I can't do number 2 as well—you know, exactly what I'm talking about!

Mind

You know enough now that you've earned some freedom with your choices, but with that freedom comes responsibility—you can't get away with lying to yourself anymore! I remember when I used to think lying to myself would get me somewhere, like when I would tell myself I was working my hardest when I was really going only halfway. Where the fuck did I think that would get me? I honestly don't know! Halfwaysville?? It certainly wasn't going to get me to my destination!

If you're going to tell yourself you're working your hardest, you better mean it. If you're lying, YOU are the only one who will pay the price of unrealized potential.

Muscle

Same as Week 19 (pages 124–126)

Week 22: Free Week

TAKE ONE WEEK OFF!!

It's that time again! After another eight weeks of hitting the weights, be sure to take this week off. Rest and recover like it's your job. Sleep in, stretch, roll it all out with some slow-ass yoga. Be good to your body.

Week 23

These last four weeks are designed for powerful aesthetic effect with a lower-body focus.

Mouth

 Here's what I'm going for this time:

Overnight Oats and Chia Bowl + Fried Eggs
Flank Steak with Sautéed Zucchini + White Rice
Kale Salad
Lamb Chops and Roasted Potatoes + Eggplant + Asparagus

 Get your 10-day check-in done on day two of this week!

Mind

I have a bad habit of looking to others for validation. For so many years, I didn't even realize I had this habit, and it seriously took me going to therapy for the first time as a full-on, (mostly) functioning adult at the age of 33. It took hours of uncomfortable, squirm-inducing one-on-one time with a near stranger for me to come to this realization.

This near stranger, my therapist, was the first person in my life to say to me, "You've got to love yourself first before you can accept love from others." Or maybe it was more like, "Quit chasing the approval of others when what you seek is your own." Really, it was probably like some kind of jumbled mix of the two—I was too busy bawling my eyes out to hear it perfectly, but I got the point. And it's a point I want to share with you: You've got to be your number one supporter, every damn day. Because at the end of the day (and the beginning of the day, and the middle of the day, and especially the middle of the night when you're wide awake and can't sleep), you are truly the only one who can always be there for you, for better or worse. Give yourself the gift of loving thoughts, directed your own way. Go all in. Love yourself like your life depends on it—because it does!

Muscle

Day One: Legs & Cardio
Hip thrusts (bodyweight, banded): 3 × 20
Squats (wide stance): 5 × 5
Goblet squats: 4 × 10
Good mornings: 4 × 10
Reverse lunges (dumbbells): 3 × 10 (each leg)
Plyo calf raises: 3 × 30
Squat-lunge-squat-lunges: 3 × 10
Sprints (treadmill or turf): 7 × 40-yard sprints or 7 sprints of 10 seconds on the treadmill

Day Two: Back & Abs
Face pulls: 3 × 20
Barbell rows (supinated grip): 5 × 10
KB single-arm rows: 4 × 10
Bent-over dumbbell rows: 4 × 10
Pull-ups (band assisted): 4 × 10
Lying leg lifts: 4 × 20
Kneeling rope crunches: 4 × 20
Sprints: 10 sprints of 15 seconds within 8 minutes

Day Three: Legs
KB dead lifts to squat: 3 × 10
Hip thrusts (bodyweight, banded): 5 × 5
Sumo squats: 5 × 10 (1-second pause at bottom)
Leg presses (wide stance): 4 × 15–20
Bulgarian split squats: 4 × 10 (each leg)
Standing calf raises: 4 × 10
Plyo split lunges: 3 × 10 (each leg)

KB pulsating squats: 3 × 30
Drop squats (banded): 3 × 20

Day Four: Hybrid
Biceps straight-bar curls: 4 × 20
Barbell drag curls: 4 × 20
Triceps cable pull-downs (rope): 4 × 20
Standing rope triceps pull-overs: 4 × 20
Assisted dips: 4 × 15
Military presses: 5 × 12–15
Arnold presses: 4 × 12–15
Lateral raises: 4 × 20

Day Five: Legs
KB swings: 3 × 20
Sumo dead lifts: 5 × 5
Dumbbell stiff-leg dead lifts: 4 × 10
KB single-leg lunges: 3 × 10 (each leg)
Hamstring curls (cable): 4 × 20
Plyo sumos: 3 × 12–20
Plyo calf raises: 3 × 30
Plyo split lunges: 3 × 8–12 (each leg)

Day Six: Active Recovery
45 minutes of foam rolling or
45-minute walk or
90-minute hot yoga class

Week 24

Mouth

✗ How are you liking the mandatory Active Recovery days? DO NOT SKIP THESE. In addition to getting in your recovery activities, make sure to eat accordingly and drink plenty of water. If you feel like you need an extra meal some days, just have it! Yup, you know the difference between "food" and nutrients now, so listen to your body and nourish it. Also, never say no to opportunities for extra sleep when they appear—your body needs rest to make progress!

 Get your 10-day check-in done on day five of this week!

Mind

Remember those goals we set out to create at the beginning? Do you remember my whole spiel about them being specific and measurable enough, yet living at the edge of realistic and ambitious? It's time you dust off these said goals. Go ahead, I'll wait right here until you bring them out into the clear.

Got them? Okay, let's assess where you're at versus the goals you set out. One by one I want you to answer these questions:

1. Were my actions from the beginning consistent with the goals that I set for myself?

2. What level of adherence have I achieved with the actions that I know will drive me toward my goals? Was it 70%, 90%, etc.? Do I feel like I can do better?

3. Are these goals in line with what I want my life to be, or do I need to reassess?

As usual, I want you to be very honest with yourself, not harsh or mean, just honest. Go back and read the answers to my questions about your goals and see if you're being honest.

.... *Mel's Tip* ....

It's not enough to just write down your goals and the things you want in life—you have to also go back and read these declarations of desire. Surprisingly, this second step is *way* harder than the first. Why is it harder? Honesty. Yup. At least for me, it's terrifying to write something down that I believe is a "must have" in my life, knowing that three months later, I might have to be confronted by the reality that I haven't done shit about it. Despite that scary reality, I've found that being honest and admitting that you haven't made good on certain promises to yourself—in instances where it's true!— is the only way to get better at following through and producing positive change.

Okay, so honesty check done. Now that you are deeply aware of where you were, where you are, and maybe even where you wish to go, let's get back to work!

Muscle

 Day One: Legs
Drop squats (banded): 3 × 20
Dead lifts: 7 × 7
Sumo dead lifts: 4 × 10
Dumbbell stiff-leg dead lifts: 4 × 10
Single-leg lying hamstring extensions: 4 × 10 (each leg)
KB pulsating sumos: 3 × 20
Plyo sumos: 3 × 12
Banded diagonal-forward crab walks: 3 × 10 (each leg)

·· *Mel's Tip* ··
Did you know you can be cute AF and bossbitch AF at the same time? Try it out! Also, this leg day—ouch. I think this one might have left me sore for about a week.
··

Day Two: Hybrid (Arms & Shoulders)
Biceps rope curls: 3 × 20
Biceps barbell curls: 4 × 15–20
Alternating biceps dumbbell curls: 3 × 12
Triceps cable push-down (straight bar): 3 × 20
Seated triceps pull-overs: 4 × 20
Dips (bodyweight): 4 × 10
Arnold presses: 3 × 12
Front raises to lateral raises: 3 × 12

Day Three: Legs
Cable glute kick-backs: 4 × 20
Squats (wide stance): 7 × 7
Front squats: 4 × 10

Quad extension machine: 4 × 20
Dumbbell static lunges: 4 × 10 (each leg)
KB single-leg lunges: 3 × 10 (each leg)
KB dead lifts to squat: 3 × 10
Plyo sumos: 3 × 10–12
Plyo split lunges: 4 × 10–12 (each leg)

Day Four: Back & Abs
Plank holds: 4 × 1 minute
Bent-over dumbbell rows: 5 × 10–15
Seated V-bar cable rows: 4 × 15–20
Cable rows: 4 × 20
Lat pull-downs (wide grip): 4 × 12–15
Lat V-bar pull-downs: 4 × 20
Hanging leg lifts: 4 × 20
Bicycle sprints: 7 sprints of 20 seconds over 10 minutes

Mel's Tip

Treat every rep like the first one, put all your focus into your workout, and have integrity in your work and progress will come, or at least be just right around the corner. Keep turning, baby!

Day Five: Legs
Squats (bodyweight): 3 × 20
Hip thrusts (barbell, banded): 7 × 7 (fluid reps)
Good mornings: 5 × 10
Single-leg lying hamstring extensions: 4 × 10 (each leg)
KB dead lifts to squats: 3 × 10–12
KB pulsating sumos: 3 × 30
Banded hamstring curls: 100 reps
Plyo sumos: 3 × 20

Day Six: Active Recovery

60-minute massage or

45-minute hot bath or

60-minute sauna

Week 25

Mind

Self-love, self-worth, and self-esteem start with the same basic ingredient: honesty. It's easy to lie—you lie to other people and even to yourself. But, if you look in the mirror and you try to say a lie out loud, it's impossible for you to believe it. You feel this in the very pit of your stomach. When you start to be honest with yourself about who you are, the real YOU and not the one you show to people, that is when you can start to be true to yourself, because then you can't put up with any other version. When you start to be honest with yourself, you can't go back. Then you start to be honest with others and demand honesty as well. This is the first step to taking control, ownership, responsibility for your life.

Muscle

Day One: Legs

Banded diagonal-forward crab walks: 3 × 10 (each leg)

Sumo dead lifts: 10 × 10

Dead lifts: 4 × 10

Dumbbell stiff-leg dead lifts: 3 × 20

Good mornings: 4 × 10

Walking lunges with dumbbells: 3 × 10 (each leg)

Plyo sumos: 3 × 20

Walking lunges (bodyweight): 3 × 12 (each leg with 1-second hold at bottom)

Squat-lunge-squat-lunges: 3 × 10

Day Two: Hybrid (Back & Chest & Abs)

KB single-arm rows: 4 × 12

Cable rows: 3 × 12–15

Lat pull-downs (wide grip): 3 × 12–15
Cable chest flies: 4 × 20
Dumbbell incline chest presses: 4 × 12–15
Hanging leg lifts: 4 × 20
Decline sit-ups: 4 × 20 (may use dumbbells for extra resistance)
Bicycle sprints: 7 sprints of 20 seconds each within 8 minutes

Day Three: Legs
Cable glute kick-backs: 3 × 50 (each leg)
Hip thrusts (barbell, banded): 10 × 10
Leg presses (wide stance): 3 × 10
Leg presses (narrow stance): 3 × 10
Hamstring curl machine: 3 × 20
KB dead lifts to squats: 3 × 10
KB pulsating sumos: 3 × 20
Plyo sumos: 3 × 12–15
Banded step-outs: 3 × 10 (each leg)

Day Four: Hybrid (Arms & Shoulders)
Biceps barbell curls: 4 × 20
Alternating biceps dumbbell curls: 4 × 10–15 (each arm)
Assisted dips: 4 × 15
Triceps cable push-downs (straight bar): 4 × 20
Triceps bent-over kick-backs: 4 × 12 (together)
Lying leg lifts: 5 × 30
Decline sit-ups: 4 × 15

Day Five: Legs
Walking lunges (bodyweight): 3 × 20 (each leg)
Squats (bodyweight): 10 × 10
Front squats: 4 × 10
Goblet squats: 4 × 10
Walking lunges with dumbbells: 4 × 12 (each leg)

Single-leg quad extensions: 4 × 10 (each leg)
Drop squats (banded): 4 × 20
KB swings: 4 × 20
Plyo split lunges: 3 × 10 (each leg)

Day Six: Active Recovery
60-minute yoga class or
45 minutes of foam rolling or
90-minute hot yoga class

Week 26

Mouth

I know you're probably like, "Mel, I GET IT, I get how to eat now." But let me suggest something to you—if there's a meal you haven't tried in the recipes, I challenge you to do that this week. Mix it up, for the sake of your taste buds.

Get your 10-day check-in done on day one of this week. Last check-in of The Turn-around! NBD. Just 26 weeks of kicking ass at taking care of yourself with real-deal nutrition.

Mind

 How are you feeling? Let me guess—you never thought your body could do shit like this. You now know what feeling strong actually feels like, and I'm not talking just physical strength. There have been ups and downs, and downs and ups, and yet you made it right to this very moment. For whatever reason, you may be feeling scared. At least that's how I felt when I was on the verge of reaching my first "finish line," and how I feel every time I'm about to wrap up a certain training plan with a clear end point.

Although you might feel like you're a pro now, you've been cruising along supported by training wheels. In addition to killing the rest of your training, I want you to take the training wheels off and actually and truly create the life that you want. It will not be easy—there's no how-to manual here, that's not how life works. I wanted to share with you how to think and do in harmony, that's been my goal. The rest is up to you; trust your gut (intuition)!

Muscle

Day One: Hybrid Legs

Squat-lunge-squat-lunges: 3 × 10
Dead lifts: 4 × 10
Dumbbell stiff-leg dead lifts: 3 × 20
Squats (wide stance): 4 × 10
Goblet squats: 3 × 20
Hip thrusts (barbell, banded): 4 × 10
Leg presses (wide stance): 3 × 20
KB dead lifts to squats: 3 × 10
KB swings: 2 × 40
Plyo sumos: 2 × 20

Day Two: Hybrid (Arms & Shoulders)

Biceps rope curls: 4 × 20
Biceps barbell curls: 4 × 12
Triceps cable pull-downs (rope): 4 × 20
Standing rope triceps pull-overs: 4 × 12
Military presses: 5 × 20
Arnold presses: 4 × 12
Lateral raises: 3 × 20
Push-ups: 3 × 10

Day Three: Hybrid Legs

Walking lunges (bodyweight): 3 × 10 (each leg, fluid)
Hip thrusts (barbell, banded): 4 × 10
Dumbbell static lunges: 3 × 12 (each leg)
Dumbbell stiff-leg dead lifts: 4 × 10
KB single-leg lunges: 3 × 10 (each leg)
Hamstring extension machine: 3 × 20–30
Hamstring curl machine: 3 × 20–30
Quad extension machine: 3 × 20–30
Bulgarian split squats: 3 × 10 (each leg)
Plyo sumos: 3 × 12

Day Four: Hybrid (Back & Cardio)
Face pulls: 4 × 20
Pull-ups (band assisted): 5 × 10–15
T-bar rows: 5 × 10 (1-second hold)
Lat V-bar pull-downs: 4 × 20
Bent-over dumbbell rows: 4 × 10–12
Stairmaster: 25 minutes at steady speed

Day Five: Hybrid Legs
Sumo dead lifts: 4 × 10
Dumbbell stiff-leg dead lifts: 3 × 20
Hip thrusts (bodyweight, banded): 4 × 10
Smith machine front squats: 3 × 20
Leg presses (wide stance): 4 × 10
Quad extension machine: 3 × 20
Goblet squats: 4 × 10
Single-leg lying hamstring extensions: 3 × 10 (each leg)
KB dead lifts to squats: 2 × 10
KB pulsating sumos: 2 × 20

Day Six: Active Recovery
45-minute walk or
60-minute massage or
90-minute hot yoga class

Conclusion

It's funny how the end of one thing only means the beginning of something else, something waiting for you right now. If you think about it, you're always a beginner, always closing one chapter and starting another. You never stop improving, not if you're actually trying to be better: being the best version of yourself is a lifelong journey.

You have to be honest with yourself so you can make the best choices for YOU! You have not changed, not the real you at least. Your legs and arms might be tighter, your food is definitely healthier and tastier, your love for yourself is larger, but the you inside of this amazing shell you've created has always been there looking for a way to get out. This was your out! You have grown and left your old shell behind, your iceberg of shit much smaller and your vision clearer. If you did this right, then you'll notice that some of your goals have changed—your priorities, your perspective. Maybe when you started you wanted to lose 20 pounds or you wanted toned arms, but what you realized was that the biggest thing you've gained from all those biceps curls, the (what felt like) never-ending minutes doing cardio or squat after firkin squat, is the knowledge of your potential, confidence, and power that you've never felt before.

After you've completed The Turnaround, you know this isn't the end but just the beginning. You are right at the beginning of your new life—a life you will create the way you want it, with things and people and feelings about yourself that will keep taking you to the next level of greatness.

Challenges and new beginnings will no longer be scary. You will face them differently, because you will not see them as obstacles but as opportunities. You have opened up to your potential—no more *I can'ts*. Having a rough day won't be as rough because you're better at handling it. You won't feel so shitty about that donut you ate because you know you don't need to get "back on track" to keeping living this lifestyle. Because having that donut IS part of your lifestyle now. It's no longer a fuck-up or glitch in the matrix. You eat it, you enjoy it, and THAT'S IT, THE END, you move on. You'll have shitty workouts and be tired, but you won't ever stop because you've created new neural pathways in your brain that won't let you give up on yourself. That trash talk is over. You left it behind with all your doubts and fears.

How much did you learn about yourself on this journey?

For me, I still feel like I'm learning every damn day. And it's not easy. But I know myself so much better than I did before I started my own fit journey. And in a way, that makes life harder—because when you know, you know you know, and you can't UNknow or fucking lie to yourself anymore!! But it also makes life *better*. There's nothing more freeing than taking responsibility for your choices for your life and not pointing the finger at everything and everyone. Yes, some excuses are valid, but they don't help you move forward. Prioritize yourself. That's why choosing YOU every time empowers you—if you can keep going, keep digging, keep doing the work. Because you are in your life, in your SELF, in a way that you weren't before. You feel it all: the good, the bad, the pain, sadness, happiness, and joy. It's all raw and it's all REAL. Be in it, for better or worse. Because you sure as shit are married to yourself for the rest of your life. No one can ever love you more than YOU. How much do you want to love yourself?

Now go read this book again.

The Turnaround Toolbox

Recipes

Well, hello there, hungry people! This section contains the recipes that aim to deliver taste, texture, and experience, and BONUS—they just happen to align with The Turnaround you're making. I could absolutely have you make and eat food that will deliver "faster" results, but at the expense of your health and sustainability—yeah, no, sorry. We're here to end the yo-yo lifestyle and create physical and mental habits that work long term.

I've organized the recipes in a super easy way by category (smoothies, salads, dinner, etc.) so you can try anything you want any day of the week and find the recipes you want to make and remake and remake again. You'll find some crowd favorites such as huevos rancheros and bibimbap, and a bunch of vegetarian options as well. Vegetarian recipes are marked (V). The reason behind this is that you don't need to live and die on a diet—quite the opposite, actually. I want you to open your mind to the endless possibilities of what nutrition can do for you.

Finally, I have a separate section called Nutrient-Rich Sides. I left this section separate from the lunch and dinner recipes because I want you to be able to choose the micronutrient source (veggies mostly), carbs, and proteins for your meals. In the food intro section, you learned how to compute your macros (protein, carbs, fat), but your body can't possibly work at its best if you don't consume the trace amounts of fiber (hugely important), vitamins, and minerals it needs; yes, you need micros for your body to break down the macros.

Also, I want you to learn to cook your veggies and other staples and develop a taste for them. You'll also be able to create your own meals by rearranging the different food groups as you see fit. You'll thank me forever, I promise!

Here are the many amazing options you have to choose from! Seriously, there is no way you won't find some forever favorites here.

Lunch/Dinner

Lamb Chops and Roasted Red Potatoes 147

Ground Turkey Kofta 149

Flank Steak with Sautéed Zucchini 150

Roasted Chicken with Peperonata..151

Salmon with Broccolini...152

Brown Rice Poke Bowl..153

Vietnamese-Style Ground Chicken Lettuce Wraps......................... 154

Whole Tandoori Roasted Chicken...155

Beef and Broccoli 156

Bibimbap...157

Green Curry Thai Coconut (V) 158

Mediterranean-Style Bean Salad (V).. 159

Green Tea Soba Noodles (V)...160

Our Favorite Grain Bowl (V)..161

Cauliflower Steak with Gremolata (V)..162

Lentil and Kale Soup (V)... 163

Nutrient-Rich Sides

Veggie Sides

Baby Spinach 1064

Broccoli..165

Kale 165

Cauliflower 166

Brussels Sprouts 167

Asparagus..167

Carb Sides

White Rice..168

Brown Rice 169

Sweet Potatoes (Japanese)...170

Eggplant..170

Protein Sides

Chicken, Beef, Fish, Tempeh, or Tofu 171

Salmon 172

Fried Eggs 172

Smoothies

Strawberry Banana 173

Green 174

Almond Butter and Berry 174

Matcha Oat 175

Salads

Kale Salad 176

Caesar (Grilled Chicken Optional) 177

Classic Niçoise 178

Cobb 179

Breakfast

Mushroom Frittata 180

Shakshuka 181

Huevos Rancheros 182

Paleo Pancakes with Blueberry Syrup 183

Overnight Oats and Chia Bowl 184

Snacks

Kale Chips 185

Egg-Salad-Stuffed Celery 186

Hummus 187

Guacamole with Sweet Potato Chips 188

Desserts

Dark Chocolate Nutty Bark..189

Blueberry Banana Pops..190

Flourless Chocolate Cake..191

Oatmeal Almond Cookies 192

Banana Chocolate Bread..193

Gluten-Free Sweet Potato Pie...194

Lamb Chops and Roasted Red Potatoes

This is a simple recipe that will impress at any dinner party. Be sure to choose a recipe from the veggies section to get your micros intake and add some green jazz to your life.

The rub is excellent for all types of meat. If not using it for lamb, I suggest trying it on chicken. Venison is also tasty with this rub!

Serve the lamb chops with the delicious mint chimichurri (aka gremolata).

SERVES 4

2 pounds rack of lamb (8 ribs)

12 baby red potatoes, sliced in half

1 to 2 teaspoons sunflower or coconut oil

Sea salt and cracked black pepper to taste

For the rub

½ cup cilantro leaves with tender stems

½ cup flat-leaf parsley leaves

½ cup mint leaves

½ tablespoon ground cumin

½ tablespoon paprika

2 teaspoons allspice

1 teaspoon crushed red pepper

2 tablespoons olive oil

1 tablespoon sea salt

For the gremolata

1 bunch mint, chopped

1 bunch parsley, chopped

2 tablespoons chives, finely chopped

2 cloves fresh garlic, minced

1 teaspoon crushed red pepper

1 tablespoon red wine vinegar

6 tablespoons olive oil

Chop all ingredients for the rub and mix with the two tablespoons of olive oil. Generously rub the rack of lamb all over and allow to marinate for about 4 hours before cooking. Remove it from refrigerator about 1 hour before you're ready to cook it to allow it to return to room temperature. (This makes for more even cooking.)

Preheat the oven to 450°F.

In a large bowl, mix the potatoes with sunflower or coconut oil, salt, and pepper. Arrange the potatoes, cut sides up, on a large baking sheet lined with foil. Set aside.

Top a separate baking sheet with a wire baking rack, and place the lamb on top of the rack. Transfer to the middle of your preheated oven, and while you have your oven open (efficiency, baby!), grab the reserved tray of potatoes and put it on the lower rack. Allow both to roast for 20 minutes.

Reduce heat to 350°F and roast lamb until done. Using a meat thermometer, check the temperature every 10 minutes, since cooking times vary depending on the oven. The USDA recommends that lamb be cooked to an internal temperature of 145°F, but I recommend removing it from the oven at 140°F—the temperature will continue to rise after it is removed. Allow the rack to rest for 20 minutes before carving.

At about 30 minutes of cooking time, the potatoes should be done. Check doneness by using a cake tester or fork to pierce the surface of the potatoes. If there is little to no resistance, remove the potatoes from the oven.

For the gremolata

Add the herbs, garlic, and red pepper to a food processor and blend for 45 seconds, or until it has a nice powder-like consistency.

Spoon the mixture into a glass jar with a lid and add the wine vinegar and olive oil. Cap tightly and shake vigorously. You may store the gremolata at room temperature for up to one week, longer if refrigerated.

Ground Turkey Kofta

This is a very versatile recipe that can be used with any of your favorite ground meats, not just turkey. Add a carb and a veggie from those respective categories and now you have a recipe that turns into 12 thousand! LOL!

SERVES 4

2 pounds ground turkey

2 shallots, finely chopped

2 cloves fresh garlic, finely chopped

1 tablespoon fresh mint, chopped

½ cup fresh parsley, chopped

½ teaspoon cumin

¾ teaspoon hot paprika

1 teaspoon cracked black pepper

1 tablespoon sea salt

2 teaspoons sunflower or coconut oil

Skewers

For the yogurt sauce

1 cup Greek yogurt

1 teaspoon sea salt

1 tablespoon fresh mint, chopped

1 tablespoon fresh parsley, chopped

1 tablespoon lemon juice

Start by making the yogurt sauce. Put all ingredients except the lemon juice in a bowl and mix with a spoon for 1 minute.

Add the lemon juice slowly while stirring the sauce. Refrigerate until ready to use.

For the kofta, combine the ground turkey in a bowl with shallots, garlic, herbs, spices, and salt and pepper. Mix until combined. Divide the seasoned meat into 2-inch logs and refrigerate for 1 hour, so they hold their shape when cooking. When the logs are firm, carefully insert skewers. Place a cast-iron pan on medium-high heat and heat the oil until it is lightly smoking. Cook the logs until they are browned, about 4 minutes on each side. Serve with yogurt sauce. Enjoy!

Flank Steak with Sautéed Zucchini

Flank steak is especially great because it is one of the leanest cuts of beef and can be very flavorful if cooked with care. You can cook flank and other steaks to your preferred doneness—here's a quick temperature guide for cooking all beefsteaks:

Rare: 125°F–130°F
Medium Rare: 130°F–135°F
Medium: 140°F–145°F
Well Done: 160°F and higher

SERVES 4

5 zucchinis, quartered lengthwise

4 teaspoons sunflower or coconut oil

Sea salt and cracked black pepper to taste

Ground garlic powder to taste

1 teaspoon dried oregano

1 teaspoon olive oil

4 tablespoons balsamic vinegar

1 pound flank steak

Put the zucchini in a bowl with the oil, salt, pepper, garlic powder, and oregano. Allow the zucchini to marinate for at least 15 minutes.

Meanwhile, heat a large cast-iron skillet slicked with oil over medium-high heat. When the pan is lightly smoking, add the zucchini. Cook for about 5 minutes, then flip it over and brush with balsamic vinegar. Cook for 3 minutes more, then flip it over once more and cook for an additional 2 minutes. Remove from the heat, slide the zucchini onto a plate, and wipe out the pan for your steaks.

Salt is important not only for flavor but also for moisture. Seasoning your steak with salt before cooking will draw out excess moisture and ensure a rich, brown crust. Your steak should always be room temperature before you begin cooking, and pat it dry. Heat the oil until it is lightly smoking. Sear the steak evenly on both sides. Your preferred doneness determines the cooking time, from 3 to 9 minutes per side.

Allow the steak to rest for 10 minutes before slicing it for serving. Resting helps retain the steak's juices.

Roasted Chicken with Peperonata

You can use any of your favorite cuts of chicken for this. I like this recipe for its ability to turn cooking one dinner into doing meal prep for a few days.

SERVES 5

½ cup sunflower or coconut oil

8 cloves garlic, crushed

3 small onions, sliced

Sea salt and cracked black pepper to taste

2 red bell peppers, seeded and sliced

2 orange bell peppers, seeded and sliced

2 yellow bell peppers, seeded and sliced

1 cup canned tomatoes or 6 very ripe tomatoes

2 sprigs basil

2 sprigs oregano

1 tablespoon red wine vinegar

5 chicken breasts

½ lemon

In a large pot, gently heat the oil. Add garlic and cook over a low flame for about 4 minutes. Stir in the onions and let them sweat for 5 minutes, until they are opaque. Season with salt. Add the sliced bell peppers and stir occasionally until cooked through. This will take about 15 minutes. Add the tomatoes, crush them up, and cook for 30 minutes. Add the basil and oregano and cook for another 15 minutes. Add the red wine vinegar and remove the peperonata from the heat.

Season chicken breasts with salt and pepper. Place them on a sheet pan lined with a rack and place it in the oven for 20 minutes. Cook until the chicken has reached 145°F; check with a meat thermometer. Remove the sheet pan from the oven and let the chicken rest for at least 10 minutes before serving.

Squeeze the lemon over the chicken and serve it with the peperonata.

Salmon with Broccolini

This is a good weeknight or weekend option, since it's simple but kinda makes you look fancy when you cook it. I like to enjoy this dish with some white rice to make sure I'm hitting all macros and micros numbers.

SERVES 3

1 pound salmon fillet, with skin

1 teaspoon + 1 tablespoon sunflower or coconut oil

Sea salt and cracked black pepper to taste

1 tablespoon pine nuts

2 bunches broccolini

2 cloves fresh garlic, minced

½ teaspoon anchovy paste

½ lemon

For the salmon

Select broil on your oven. Rub the salmon lightly on all sides with 1 teaspoon oil and season with salt and pepper. Place salmon with skin side up on the highest rack of your oven. Broil for 10 minutes. Switch to the "bake" setting on your oven. Remove the salmon from the oven, and turn it over. Bake on a middle rack of the oven for 10 minutes.

For the pine nuts

Spread the pine nuts on a baking tray and put it in the preheated oven. Shake the tray every five minutes to ensure even toasting. When the pine nuts are toasted to your liking, remove from the oven and season with a little salt.

For the broccolini

Cut the broccolini into individual stalks, removing any woody ends. Heat 1 tablespoon oil in a skillet. Place the broccolini in the pan and cook for 4 minutes, then flip it over. Add garlic and anchovy paste and stir the broccolini to fully incorporate the seasonings. Cook for another 4 minutes and remove from heat. Squeeze the lemon over it and sprinkle with toasted pine nuts.

Brown Rice Poke Bowl

This recipe is very simple, quick, and refreshing. One pro tip: Replace ½ cup of water with rice wine vinegar for cooking the rice. This will add a nice flavor and great texture to the rice.

SERVES 2

8 ounces sushi-grade tuna,
    cut into small, bite-size cubes

Sea salt to taste

2 tablespoons rice vinegar

1 teaspoon sesame oil

1 cup cooked brown rice

3 scallions, thinly sliced

2 radishes, thinly sliced

1 English cucumber, thinly sliced

¼ avocado, thinly sliced

1 teaspoon sesame seeds

In a large bowl, season the tuna with salt, rice vinegar, and oil. Remove from bowl and set aside, reserving the liquid.

Divide the rice into two bowls and top with tuna. Add vegetables and avocado, and pour any remaining liquid over the top. Sprinkle everything with sesame seeds. Enjoy!

Vietnamese-Style Ground Chicken Lettuce Wraps

A little bit of sauce goes a long way! You can stretch about two tablespoons of sauce for your whole meal.

SERVES 2

1 tablespoon sunflower or coconut oil

10 ounces ground chicken

3 cloves fresh garlic, minced

1 stalk lemongrass, tough outer layers removed, lower 6 inches of tender bulb, finely chopped

4 scallions, thinly sliced

1 tablespoon fresh ginger, grated

Sea salt and cracked black pepper to taste

2 teaspoons fish sauce

2 heads Boston lettuce, separated into single leaves

½ bunch fresh mint, leaves picked

½ bunch fresh cilantro, leaves picked

½ bunch fresh Thai basil, leaves picked

For the sauce

3 limes, juiced

4 tablespoons fish sauce

1 tablespoon rice vinegar

4 tablespoons honey

¼ cup water

Pinch of crushed red pepper

Add the oil to a large skillet. Add the ground chicken, garlic, lemongrass, scallions, ginger, salt, and pepper to the pan and stir to mix the ingredients thoroughly. Continue to stir and break apart the ground chicken, cooking for about 10 minutes or until the meat is no longer pink. Add the splash of fish sauce and stir for another minute. Remove the contents from the skillet.

For the sauce, in a medium-size bowl, whisk together the lime juice, fish sauce, rice vinegar, and honey. Whisk in the water and crushed red pepper.

Assemble the lettuce wraps with the herbs of your choice. Lightly dip each wrap in the sauce. Enjoy!

Whole Tandoori Roasted Chicken

Roasting a whole chicken is awesome because it 1) saves you money, and 2) gives you the most juicy and delicious chicken ever! Don't think you have to go for the breasts just because they have fewer calories—my favorite parts of the chicken are actually the legs and wings. Enjoy whichever parts are your preference!

SERVES 6

For the marinade

4 tablespoons fresh ginger, grated

1 whole head fresh garlic, peeled and minced

1 tablespoon ground cumin

1 tablespoon ground coriander

1 tablespoon sweet paprika

2 teaspoons garam masala

1 teaspoon ground fenugreek

2 teaspoons harissa or red chili paste

1 lemon, juiced

4 tablespoons olive oil

3 pounds roaster chicken (approx. 2)

For the sauce

½ cup 2% Greek yogurt

½ English cucumber, julienned

1 lemon, juiced

Sea salt and cracked black pepper to taste

Whisk all the marinade ingredients together and rub the whole chicken with your marinade liquid. Don't forget to rub the inside of the chicken as well. Cover and let marinate in the refrigerator overnight or for at least 6 hours.

Remove the chicken from the fridge and preheat the oven to 350°F. Once the chicken is at room temperature, place it in a baking pan and put it in the oven (the pan will catch the juices as the chicken cooks). Roast until the internal temperature reaches 165°F, about 60 to 75 minutes. Baste the chicken with the marinade juices every 10 minutes.

Meanwhile, in a medium bowl, whisk together the Greek yogurt, julienned cucumber, and lemon juice. Season with salt and pepper to taste.

Remove the chicken from the oven and let it rest for 20 minutes before serving. Serve with yogurt sauce and your favorite naan or brown rice (just be sure to add your choice of carb to your total macros).

Beef and Broccoli

Easy, delicious, and portable. What else can you ask for? I recommend adding some brown rice from the carb recipes in order to make this a bullet-proof meal of go-to goodness.

SERVES 5

1 tablespoon sunflower or coconut oil

24 ounces sirloin steak, cut into thin slices

2 heads broccoli, cut into bite-size florets

3 cloves fresh garlic, minced

1 tablespoon soy sauce

½ teaspoon sesame seeds

½ teaspoon crushed red pepper

1 teaspoon sesame oil, for finishing

1 lime, juiced, for finishing

Heat oil in a skillet over medium heat. Once the pan starts lightly smoking, add the sirloin steak slices and cook for about 2 minutes until browned, then flip each slice and cook for another 2 minutes. Remove from the pan and set aside.

In the same pan, add the broccoli florets, heads facing down, stems up. Cook for 4 minutes, then flip, stir, and cook for another 4 minutes.

Add the cooked sirloin slices back to the skillet with the broccoli. Add garlic, soy sauce, sesame seeds, and crushed red pepper. Stir and cook for about 2 minutes, then finish the mixture with a drizzle of sesame oil and freshly squeezed lime juice.

Serve over a bed of brown rice or quinoa (about ½ cup per serving—just be sure to add your choice of carb to your total macros).

Bibimbap

This dish is great because each ingredient can be prepped in bulk and used throughout the week.

SERVES 4

2 cups cooked brown rice

4 cups bean sprouts

4 cups spinach

Sea salt to taste

1 large carrot, julienned and lightly salted

1 tablespoon sunflower or coconut oil

2 cups shiitake mushrooms, thinly sliced

1 pound lean ground beef

2 cloves fresh garlic

2 teaspoons fresh ginger, grated

1 tablespoon low-sodium soy sauce

4 tablespoons Korean red pepper paste

2 tablespoons rice vinegar

4 eggs, fried in ½ teaspoon sunflower or coconut oil (optional)

Fill a large pot halfway with water. Lightly season the water with salt. Bring to a boil and add the bean sprouts in a metal strainer. (This way, you can remove the sprouts without discarding the boiling water.) Blanch for 3 minutes. Transfer the sprouts to a large bowl of ice water to shock them and stop them from cooking. Strain and set aside.

Do the same with the spinach. Once it is blanched and shocked, set it aside.

Arrange the carrot slices on a plate and lightly salt. Let the salt draw out some moisture for at least 20 minutes as it seasons the carrot slices.

Add ½ tablespoon oil to a large skillet over medium-high heat. When the pan is lightly smoking, add the sliced shiitake mushrooms and let them cook for about 2 minutes. Lightly season with sea salt and stir to ensure even cooking. Remove mushrooms from the pan.

Add another ½ tablespoon oil to the pan. When the pan is hot, add the lean ground beef, garlic, and freshly grated ginger. Cook for about 10 minutes, stirring occasionally while breaking the meat apart. Once it is browned and fully cooked, add the low-sodium soy sauce. Remove from heat.

In a small bowl, whisk together the red pepper paste with the rice wine vinegar to create a thick sauce. Set aside.

Assemble all the vegetables over a bowl of hot brown rice. Top it off with the cooked beef and fried egg (optional) and the red pepper sauce. You can add as much of the sauce as you'd like. It's spicy, so start off with a little bit!

Green Curry Thai Coconut (V)

This is a great recipe for when you're feeling like Thai food in the comfort of your own home. The cool thing about this recipe is that you can add whatever protein or veggie from either of those sections if you want to convert it to non-vegetarian and have the complete restaurant experience that fits your macros. This recipe is best enjoyed among friends and family.

SERVES 4

1 can coconut milk

1 tablespoon green curry paste

½ bunch fresh cilantro

4 sprigs fresh basil, stemmed

1 tablespoon fresh ginger, grated

1 small eggplant, cut into 2-inch-thick medallions

1 zucchini, cut into 2-inch-thick medallions

1 green bell pepper, cut into bite-size pieces

1 cup button mushrooms, quartered

1 cup green beans, cut in half

1 small white onion, thinly sliced

1 tablespoon sunflower or coconut oil

Combine the coconut milk, curry paste, cilantro, basil, and ginger in a blender and blend until smooth. Set the curry aside.

Combine all the vegetables in a large skillet with the oil and cook for about 5 minutes over medium-high heat. Add the curry to the pan, bring to a boil, and reduce the heat to a slow simmer. Simmer the mixture for about 15 minutes or until the vegetables are tender.

Serve over brown rice (see my Brown Rice recipe from the carbs section).

Mediterranean-Style Bean Salad (V)

Another easy and simple vegetarian-inspired recipe that delivers a fresh summer vibe; it gives me a 100%-summer-in-California feeling. Add your favorite greens such as raw baby spinach, romaine lettuce, kale, etc., and get the fiber and micros you crave.

SERVES 4

1 can black beans, drained and rinsed

1 can white beans, drained and rinsed

1 red onion, diced

1 English cucumber, thinly sliced

1 cup cherry tomatoes, halved

½ cup Greek olives, pitted and halved

¼ cup feta cheese (optional)

2 tablespoons red wine vinegar

2 tablespoons olive oil

Mix all ingredients in a large bowl. Enjoy it with or without a slice of multigrain bread.

Green Tea Soba Noodles (V)

My daughter loves noodles—hence, this recipe. It's not complicated and can easily be modified to include tempeh, tofu—see the proteins section—and even chicken if you wish to depart from the vegetarian route. Hope you enjoy it as much as Bella does.

SERVES 4

16-ounce package green tea soba noodles

5 cloves fresh garlic, grated

2 tablespoons fresh ginger, grated

1 tablespoon shio dashi

1 tablespoon rice vinegar

1 teaspoon sesame oil

3 scallions, thinly sliced

1 English cucumber, julienned

½ teaspoon gochugaru (Korean ground red pepper)

4 soft-boiled eggs (optional)

Bring a large pot of water to a boil. Cook the soba noodles for about 10 minutes. When they are cooked through, strain from the pot and shock in an ice-water bath. Once the noodles have cooled down, strain from the ice water and place them in the refrigerator for 12 hours. (This not only improves their texture but makes them easier to digest.)

When you're ready to eat, mix the noodles with all the ingredients in a large bowl. Transfer to four small bowls and enjoy!

Our Favorite Grain Bowl (V)

You can bulk-prep each ingredient and make enough bowls for the whole week. This recipe is very versatile and should change from season to season. Replace the vegetables frequently with your favorites so you don't get bored! Brussels sprouts, bell peppers, and asparagus are also great additions to this bowl.

SERVES 4

1 sweet potato, diced

1 tablespoon sunflower or coconut oil

1 head broccoli, cut into bite-size florets

1 zucchini, sliced in 2-inch medallions

Sea salt and cracked black pepper to taste

1 bunch kale, sliced thin

2 cups cooked quinoa

1 cup cooked wheat berries

¼ avocado, diced (optional)

1 teaspoon red wine vinegar

½ tablespoon olive oil

Preheat the oven to 400°F. Arrange the diced sweet potato evenly on a baking sheet. You can toss it with 1 teaspoon of oil, if you like. Otherwise, just season with a little salt. Place the baking sheet in the oven and cook for about 30 minutes. Check to see if the potatoes are ready by inserting a fork or cake tester. When they are tender, remove from the heat and set aside.

Heat 1 tablespoon of oil in a large skillet over medium heat. Add the broccoli florets, heads facing down, stems up. Cook for 4 minutes and stir, then cook for another 4 minutes. Season with salt and pepper. Remove from the pan and add the zucchini slices. Cook on one side for 3 minutes, then flip to cook on the other side for another 3 minutes. Season with salt and pepper.

While the vegetables are hot, mix them in a large bowl with the raw sliced kale. This will help wilt the kale, making it soft and easier to consume. Scoop a full cup of this vegetable mixture and serve it over your quinoa and wheat berries. You can add the avocado (if using) and red wine vinegar and olive oil as a dressing. A little bit goes a long way!

Cauliflower Steak with Gremolata (V)

I really like cauliflower made this way because you can easily add some white rice and tempeh to make a full meal while keeping the cauliflower as the star of the dish. Yup, you can make cauliflower e.x.c.i.t.i.n.g!

SERVES 2

1 head cauliflower

1 teaspoon sunflower or coconut oil (for slicking the pan)

1 lemon, juiced

6 tablespoons olive oil

1 bunch fresh parsley, picked and chopped

2 tablespoons fresh chives, finely chopped

2 cloves fresh garlic, minced

1 tablespoon capers

1 teaspoon crushed red pepper

1 tablespoon red wine vinegar

Sea salt and cracked black pepper to taste

Cut cauliflower top to bottom into 3 even pieces, or "steaks," making sure the stem is holding the shape of the cauliflower together.

FOR THE GREMOLATA: In a bowl, mix together the lemon juice, olive oil, parsley, chives, garlic, capers, crushed red pepper, and red wine vinegar. Season the gremolata with salt and pepper to taste.

Heat a cast-iron pan until it is smoking hot. Add a slick of sunflower or coconut oil to the pan and let it spread evenly. Place the cauliflower in the pan, one cut face down, and allow it to sear for 4 minutes, then flip it so the other face can sear as well. The edges of the cauliflower should be almost blackened, but the inside will not be overcooked. This way, you still get all the nutrients from the vegetable.

Serve with the gremolata (for a variation, see my gremolata instructions from the Lamb Chops and Roasted Red Potatoes recipe, page 147)—and enjoy!

Lentil and Kale Soup (V)

This is for one of those days when you need something nice and warm to make you feel better or when it's just so damn cold where you live. I lived in NYC most of my life, so a little warm soup when it's 10°F outside is a welcome break. You can easily make this and pack it to take to work or school, or you can even drink it in a thermal sippy cup.

SERVES 4

1 tablespoon sunflower or coconut oil

1 medium onion, diced

1 medium carrot, diced

3 stalks celery, diced

5 cloves fresh garlic, grated

1 14-ounce can whole tomatoes

2 cups green lentils, rinsed

2 quarts vegetable stock (or water)

1 tablespoon sweet paprika

1 bunch kale, thinly sliced

Sea salt and cracked black pepper to taste

1 lemon, juiced

Add the oil to a large pot. Sweat the onions, carrots, celery, and garlic for about 5 minutes. Add the tomatoes and crush them into the vegetable mixture. When the tomatoes are fully broken up, add the lentils and 1 to 2 quarts of vegetable stock, depending on desired consistency. Bring the stock to a boil and reduce to a simmer, then add the paprika. Cook for about 30 minutes, stirring occasionally, and add the kale. Season to taste with salt and pepper. If you want soup with a looser consistency, add more vegetable stock or water. Add a squeeze of lemon juice and enjoy!

NUTRIENT-RICH SIDES

These are no-frills, superfast recipes for cooking up some seriously nutritious sides. When short on fat for the day, feel free to add some extra olive oil on your veggies once they're cooked.

VEGGIE SIDES

Baby Spinach

1 teaspoon sunflower or coconut oil

1 bunch baby spinach

Pinch of sea salt

Heat a pan (ideally cast-iron) over medium-high heat until it starts smoking a tiny bit.

Add the oil and let it heat up to pan temperature, about 30 seconds.

Add the baby spinach and stir constantly for 2 to 3 minutes.

Remove from pan, sprinkle with salt, and enjoy.

Broccoli

1 teaspoon sunflower or coconut oil
1 head broccoli

Pinch of sea salt
½ lime

Heat a pan (ideally cast-iron) over medium-high heat until it starts smoking a tiny bit.

Add the oil and let it heat up to pan temperature, about 30 seconds.

Add the broccoli, sprinkle with salt, and move it around every 30 seconds for about 5 minutes.

Cover and cook for about 2 minutes.

Remove cover and cook for another minute; remove from pan.

Squeeze lime over the broccoli and enjoy!

Kale

1 teaspoon sunflower or coconut oil
1 bunch kale, cut

½ lime

Heat a pan (ideally cast-iron) over medium-high heat until it starts smoking a tiny bit.

Add the oil and let it heat up to pan temperature, about 30 seconds.

Add the kale and stir constantly for 2 to 3 minutes.

Allow the kale to cook for another 3 to 5 minutes, depending on how tender you like it.

Remove from pan and squeeze the lime on it.

Cauliflower

½ tablespoon sunflower or coconut oil

1 head cauliflower, cored and cut into florets

Pinch of sea salt

½ lime (optional)

1 bunch cilantro, chopped (optional)

Heat a pan (ideally cast-iron) over medium-high heat until it starts smoking a tiny bit.

Add the oil and let it heat up to pan temperature, about 30 seconds.

Add the cauliflower and move it around every minute for about 5 minutes.

Cover the cauliflower and continue cooking for about 4 more minutes.

Cook uncovered for another 1 to 2 minutes and remove from pan.

Sprinkle sea salt over the cauliflower.

Optional: Once the cauliflower has cooled slightly, finish with freshly squeezed lime juice and chopped cilantro.

Brussels Sprouts

1 bunch brussels sprouts, halved

2 tablespoons sunflower or coconut oil
   (use spray bottle)

Pinch of sea salt

Heat a pan (ideally cast-iron) over medium heat until it starts smoking a tiny bit.

Spray the pan with a bit of oil and let it heat up to pan temperature, about 30 seconds.

Add the brussels sprouts, cut sides down, and allow them to cook for about 10 minutes, uncovered.

Spray with oil, turn over the brussels sprouts one by one, and allow them to cook, pressed down—I recommend using a heavy pot—for 8 to10 minutes.

Turn them once more and let them get nice and dark over medium-low heat for 3 to 5 minutes.

Sprinkle with salt. Done.

Asparagus

1 tablespoon sunflower or coconut oil

1 pound asparagus, trimmed

Pinch of sea salt

½ lime

Heat a pan (ideally cast-iron) over medium-high heat until it starts smoking a tiny bit.

Add the oil and let it heat up to pan temperature, about 30 seconds.

Add the trimmed asparagus, sprinkle with salt, and stir every 30 seconds for about 5 minutes.

Cook, covered, for about 1 minute.

Uncover and cook for about another minute; remove from pan.

Squeeze the lime over the asparagus.

When short on carbs for the day, feel free to add one of these guys to your meals. You may choose one over the other, or from the Nutrient-Rich Sides list, depending on how calorically dense you want your carbs to be. For example, white rice is more calorically dense than broccoli, but they can both be used to complete your carbs for the day. If you're short by 20 grams, for example, you may choose to go with rice, whereas you'd probably go for the broccoli if you need only 10 grams. My personal favorite is eggplant!

White Rice

1 cup white rice
Pinch of sea salt

1 teaspoon sunflower or coconut oil

Rinse the rice.

Boil some water in a pot with a lid over medium-low heat. You don't need to be super precise about the amount of water— just make sure it's enough to cover the rice.

Add the rice, removing any water beyond barely covering the surface of the rice (anything above a quarter inch).

Add the salt and oil and stir the rice with a spoon.

Let it boil, uncovered, until you see air bubbles appear all over the rice and the surface water has evaporated.

Reduce the heat to low and cook, covered, for 10 minutes. Turn the rice over with a spoon, making sure to get under the bottom.

Continue cooking, covered, for 10 minutes. Done.

Optional: You can use a rice cooker and just press the "white rice" button. The same water, oil, and salt measurements will work.

Brown Rice

1 cup brown rice   1 teaspoon sunflower or coconut oil
Pinch of sea salt

Rinse the rice.

Boil some water in a pot with a lid over medium-low heat. You don't need to be super precise about the amount of water— just make sure it's enough to cover the rice.

Add the rice, removing any water beyond barely covering the surface of the rice (anything above 1 inch).

Add the salt and oil and stir the rice with a spoon.

Let it boil, uncovered, until you see air bubbles appear all over the rice and the surface water has evaporated.

Reduce the heat to low and cook, covered, for 20 minutes. Turn the rice over with a spoon, making sure to get under the bottom.

Cook, covered, for another 10 to 15 minutes. (Check to see if it's done enough for your taste). Done.

Optional: You can use a rice cooker and just press the "brown rice" button. The same water, oil, and salt measurements will work.

Sweet Potatoes (Japanese)

1 large sweet potato

Pinch of sea salt

1 tablespoon sunflower or coconut oil

Boil sweet potato with skin on over medium-high heat for about 15 minutes. You should be able to pierce it with a fork with some resistance, but not so much that it feels raw.

Let the potato cool for about 10 minutes in the freezer, then cut it into medallions or fries (whatever shape you like).

Heat a cast-iron pan, add ½ tablespoon oil, and proceed to pan-fry the potatoes for about 8 minutes over medium-high heat.

Sprinkle the potatoes with another ½ tablespoon oil, turn them over, and pan-fry for another 8 minutes.

Let the potatoes dry on a rack, or on your plate. Don't forget to sprinkle them with some sea salt.

Eggplant

1 large eggplant

Pinch of sea salt

1 teaspoon sunflower or coconut oil (use spray bottle)

Preheat the oven to 375°F.

Cut the eggplant, with the peel on, into medallions about ¼-inch thick or fries, whatever you prefer.

Place the eggplant on a baking sheet and spray it with oil on both sides.

Place the eggplant in the oven, turning it over after 20 minutes, and continue roasting for another 20 minutes.

Remove from the oven and sprinkle with sea salt.

Chicken, Beef, Fish, Tempeh, or Tofu

This is my go-to preparation method for your favorite protein sources and it can be used to create entirely new meals using the micros + carbs recipes. You can also easily complete any macros you may be missing.

SERVES 2 OR 3

1 pound chicken, beef, fish, tempeh, or tofu

Pinch of sea salt

1 tablespoon olive oil

1 bunch cilantro, chopped

½ head fresh garlic, minced

1 tablespoon soy sauce

1 plastic freezer bag, half-gallon size

Cut 1 pound (16 ounces) of your favorite protein source into strips.

Put the strips with all the other ingredients in the plastic freezer bag and shake for 30 seconds. (Make sure to seal the bag tightly, LOL!)

Marinate for at least 24 hours before cooking.

Heat a cast-iron pan over medium-high heat for about 5 minutes.

Add the strips one by one. Let them cook for 5 to 8 minutes and flip over.

Allow to cook on the other side for another 5 to 8 minutes.

Remove from the pan and cool for about 3 minutes before serving.

Salmon

SERVES 4

1 pound wild Alaskan salmon

1 teaspoon sunflower or coconut oil

Pinch of sea salt

1 tablespoon chopped cilantro

½ lime

Rub salmon with oil and sprinkle with salt.

Heat a cast-iron pan over medium-high heat about 5 minutes.

Place salmon in the pan and allow it to cook for 8 to 10 minutes, then gently turn over.

Allow to cook on the other side for another 8 to 10 minutes.

Remove from the pan and let it cool for about 5 minutes, then sprinkle with cilantro and a squeeze of lime.

Fried Eggs

SERVES 1

3 large eggs

½ teaspoon sunflower or coconut oil

Pinch of sea salt

Slick a cast-iron pan with oil and heat over medium-high heat for about 5 minutes.

Carefully crack open one egg; you'll repeat this process 3 times.

Cook the eggs until the bottoms turn golden brown, about 3 minutes.

Carefully flip the eggs and cook for about 1 minute for a medium temperature of the yolk.

Done!

SMOOTHIES

All of your smoothie ingredients can be purchased fresh, and this way you know all the ingredients are fully washed because you wash them yourself. It's fun! You can prep your own fresh fruit and freeze it for use later. Using frozen fruit will limit your need for ice cubes, which can eventually water down the flavor of your smoothies.

Strawberry Banana

Very simple smoothie for when you want to start your day light or end it light.

SERVES 2

1 cup strawberries, washed and frozen

1 whole banana, sliced and frozen

¼ cup plain Greek yogurt or protein powder

1 tablespoon chia seeds

¼ cup raw almonds

2 cups unsweetened almond milk

Combine all the ingredients in a blender and blend until smooth. Add more almond milk if needed to create the consistency you desire.

Green

I like this one in the middle of the afternoon or right after a hard workout—it just feels right and digests well.

SERVES 2

½ cup kale, washed and frozen

½ cup spinach, washed and frozen

¼ cup raw walnuts, frozen

⅛ avocado, frozen

1 tablespoon chia seeds

1 tablespoon golden flaxseeds

¼ cup Greek yogurt or protein powder

2 cups unsweetened almond milk

Combine all the ingredients in a blender and blend until smooth. Add more almond milk if needed to create the consistency you desire.

Almond Butter and Berry

This is a crowd favorite and you can drink it or pour it into a bowl and eat it with a spoon, which is my daughter's favorite way to enjoy it!

SERVES 2

1 whole banana, sliced and frozen

1 cup blueberries, washed and frozen

2 tablespoons almond butter (or peanut butter)

2 cups unsweetened oat milk

1 tablespoon golden flaxseed

Combine all the ingredients in a blender and blend until smooth. Add more oat milk if needed to create the consistency you desire. Feel free to add protein powder to this smoothie.

Matcha Oat

If you find that this smoothie isn't cold enough, you can freeze the yogurt into small ice cube trays and use those instead of refrigerated yogurt.

SERVES 2

1 whole banana, sliced and frozen

½ cup Greek yogurt or protein powder

½ cup kale, washed and frozen

¼ cup raw oats

1 teaspoon matcha green tea powder (ceremonial grade)

2 cups unsweetened oat milk

Combine all the ingredients in a blender and blend until smooth. Add more oat milk if needed to create the consistency you desire.

SALADS

Salad doesn't necessarily equal a full meal, despite what many diets and salad bars want you to believe. That being said, a salad is potentially a nice way to add micronutrients and freshness to your palate. I like adding salad to my full meals or having some salad in the middle of the afternoon between lunch and dinner. Get wild!

Kale Salad

This is my go-to when I want to hit my micros intake and do so in style! Yup, I like kale, but I love it in this form. ;)

SERVES 2

1 bunch lacinato kale, sliced into bite-size pieces

1 small red onion, sliced thin

½ avocado, diced

½ cucumber, sliced thin

1 breakfast radish, sliced thin

¼ cup cherry tomatoes, halved

3 tablespoons pumpkin seeds, roasted or raw

1 lemon, juiced

2 tablespoons olive oil

Sea salt and cracked black pepper to taste

Throw all the ingredients except the last three in a large bowl. Put on a glove (or not!) and use your hands to thoroughly mix in the lemon juice and olive oil. Add salt and pepper to taste.

It's important to spend time massaging the kale to make it easier to digest. You'll see that as you massage the leaves, they get wilted and become a softer texture. Try not to crush the avocados as you're mixing, but it's okay if you do—they're still so delicious!

Caesar (Grilled Chicken Optional)

A classic with a twist. This one hits a home run when it comes to flavor-to-work ratio, aka easy to make, tastes really good.

SERVES 4

4 chicken breasts, grilled (optional)

Sea salt and cracked black pepper to taste

3 anchovy fillets, drained and minced

2 cloves fresh garlic, grated

1 teaspoon Dijon mustard

1 lemon, juiced

2 tablespoons red wine vinegar

¼ cup olive oil

2 slices multigrain or whole wheat bread, diced into croutons

4 romaine hearts, cut into bite-size pieces

Parmesan cheese, finely grated for serving

If you are using chicken in your salad, obviously cook it first! Season the chicken breasts with salt and pepper. Grill for 6 minutes on each side, or until they are cooked through (have reached an internal temperature of 165°F). If you do not have access to a grill, you can cook the chicken in a cast-iron pan for the same amount of time.

For the dressing, combine the anchovies, garlic, Dijon, lemon juice, and red wine vinegar in a bowl. Thoroughly whisk all ingredients and then slowly drizzle in the olive oil while continuing to whisk. Add a good amount of cracked black pepper to the dressing. I suggest using about 2 tablespoons of dressing per salad.

Preheat the oven to 325°F. Line a baking sheet with foil and spread the diced bread pieces evenly around the sheet. Place the baking sheet in the oven and toast for about 20 minutes or until the cubes are dried out. Season with salt and set aside.

Assemble by placing the romaine lettuce in a bowl and adding the chicken, croutons, and Parmesan cheese. Drizzle dressing on the salad and enjoy!

Classic Niçoise

You're absolutely going to love this salad, thanks to its flavor profile and classic French touch. I recommend you make it on a sunny Saturday afternoon.

SERVES 4

1 pound haricot verts (green beans), trimmed

1 pound small red potatoes

1 cup cherry tomatoes, quartered

½ cup pitted Niçoise olives

4 hard-boiled eggs, peeled and sliced

1 head Boston lettuce, leaves separated

1 can Italian or Spanish tuna, drained

½ shallot, minced (about 2 tablespoons)

2 tablespoons red wine vinegar

¼ cup olive oil

Sea salt and cracked black pepper to taste

Bring a large pot of water to a boil. Season with enough salt to taste like sea water. Add the trimmed haricot verts and cook for about 3 minutes. Strain the beans from the pot and shock in the ice-water bath. Set aside. In the same pot of boiling water, add the potatoes and cook for 10 to 15 minutes or until tender when poked with a fork. Remove from water and allow to cool for at least 10 minutes before cutting in half.

FOR THE DRESSING: Place the minced shallot in a bowl and add the red wine vinegar. Whisk in the olive oil and season with salt and pepper to taste. Dress each component (haricot verts, potatoes, cherry tomatoes, olives, and eggs) separately with the dressing.

Arrange all of the vegetables on a bed of Boston lettuce and top with the eggs and tuna. Enjoy!

Cobb

Just like its Caesar cousin, the Cobb is a classic and simple little salad that gives you all kinds of nostalgic vibes and tastes great!

SERVES 4

4 chicken breasts, grilled (optional)

4 romaine hearts, sliced into bite-size pieces

4 hard-boiled eggs, peeled and quartered

4 strips Canadian bacon (or turkey bacon)

1 cup cherry tomatoes, halved

1 avocado, diced

2 tablespoons chives, thinly cut

3 tablespoons red wine vinegar

5 tablespoons olive oil

1 tablespoon Dijon mustard

Sea salt and cracked black pepper to taste

Season the chicken breasts with salt and pepper. Grill for 6 minutes on each side, or until they are cooked through (have reached an internal temperature of 165°F). If you do not have access to a grill, you can cook the chicken in a cast-iron pan for the same amount of time.

Preheat the oven to 350°F. Line a baking sheet with foil and place the Canadian bacon or turkey bacon on it. Make sure there is space between the strips. Place the sheet tray in the oven and allow to cook for 20 minutes, or until completely cooked through. Remove from heat and chop the bacon into small pieces.

FOR THE DRESSING: In a bowl, whisk together the red wine vinegar, olive oil, and Dijon mustard. Season with salt and pepper to your liking.

Assemble the salad by placing the lettuce at the bottom of the plate and add each ingredient in rows. Drizzle the dressing over the salad and enjoy!

Mushroom Frittata

If you check out my stories on Insta, then you will know that I'm a fan of eggs. This frittata recipe is really good for when you want something with oomph, but you don't want to spend an hour in the kitchen. Be sure to pair it with a carb and veggie from those recipe sections to get the full meal experience.

SERVES 4

8 large eggs

¼ cup unsweetened oat milk

Sea salt and cracked black pepper to taste

1 tablespoon sunflower or coconut oil

½ cup shiitake mushrooms, sliced

½ cup oyster mushrooms, sliced

1 small white onion, diced

Preheat the oven to 400°F.

In a large bowl, whisk together eggs, oat milk, salt, and pepper. Set aside.

Add the oil to a large cast-iron skillet (or any oven-safe skillet) over medium-high heat. Once the pan is lightly smoking, add the sliced mushrooms. Cook for 1 minute and then stir so all sides can cook evenly. Add onions and cook for another 2 minutes. Season with salt and pepper.

When the mushrooms are ready, carefully pour the egg mixture into the skillet, making sure to distribute it evenly. Put the skillet in the oven and cook for about 10 minutes, or until the top and edges are golden brown.

Cool the frittata, then slice and enjoy! Frittatas freeze very well and can easily be reheated in the oven and enjoyed for up to one week.

Shakshuka

You can add crushed red pepper to this dish if you enjoy extra spice. If you don't want to turn on the oven to finish this dish, that's okay! Just close your skillet with a lid and leave it on the stovetop (definitely the better option on hot days).

SERVES 2

2 tablespoons sunflower or coconut oil

1 yellow onion, diced

1 red bell pepper, diced

4 cloves fresh garlic, grated

2 tablespoons concentrated tomato paste

1 teaspoon ground coriander

1 teaspoon ground cumin

1 teaspoon sweet paprika

1 28-ounce can whole tomatoes

Sea salt and cracked black pepper to taste

6 large eggs

1 tablespoon parsley, finely chopped, for garnish

Multigrain bread or whole-wheat pita, for serving

Preheat oven to 400°F.

Add the oil to a hot skillet over medium heat. Sweat the onion, bell pepper, and garlic for about 2 minutes, stirring occasionally to make sure all sides are cooked, but not over-cooked. Add the tomato paste and allow the vegetables to absorb it for about 2 minutes, or until the color turns to brick-red. Add the coriander, cumin, and sweet paprika and stir. Mix in the tomatoes and crush them as they heat up. Once they're fully crushed, bring the contents of the skillet to a quick boil and reduce to a simmer for about 5 minutes. Season the stewed vegetables with salt and pepper to your liking.

Using a spoon, create 6 evenly spread wells in the vegetable mixture. Crack an egg into each well. Pop the skillet into the oven for about 10 minutes. If you do not wish to use an oven, you can simply cover the skillet and continue to cook on the stovetop over low heat for another 10 minutes.

Once the eggs are done to your liking, remove and sprinkle with parsley. Enjoy with multigrain bread or whole-wheat pita.

Huevos Rancheros

I'm not going to lie: You are going to like this recipe and end up basically eating it for breakfast every day for the next two years of your life. Yup, it's that good.

SERVES 4

2 large ripe tomatoes, diced

3 small red onions, diced

¼ bunch cilantro, chopped

Sea salt and cracked black pepper to taste

2 limes, juiced

2 tablespoons sunflower or coconut oil

1 can black beans, rinsed and drained

1 teaspoon ground cumin

4 eggs

4 corn tortillas

1 avocado, thinly sliced

Salsa, if desired

FOR THE PICO DE GALLO: Mix the tomatoes, dice of two of the red onions, and cilantro in a bowl. Season with salt, pepper, and lime juice. Set the pico aside.

Heat 1 tablespoon of the oil in a skillet over medium heat. When the pan is lightly smoking, add the black beans, dice of the remaining red onion, and cumin. Stir occasionally and cook for about 10 minutes.

In a separate pan, heat the remaining 1 tablespoon of oil over medium heat. Fry the four eggs sunny-side up. When they are cooked to your liking, season with salt and pepper and remove from heat.

Assemble by placing the corn tortillas on a plate, filling them with the hot beans and pico de gallo. Add one egg to each plate and top them off with a couple slices of avocado and your favorite salsa!

Paleo Pancakes with Blueberry Syrup

The people's champ! Yup, I love pancakes that much. The best thing about this recipe is that it has a high packability and portability—that way you can enjoy it when and where you like it. The more you make these pancakes, the better they come out—I guarantee it!

SERVES 2

1 cup almond flour

¼ cup tapioca flour

¼ cup coconut flour

1 teaspoon baking powder

1 teaspoon sea salt

4 large eggs

¼ cup unsweetened oat milk

1 teaspoon pure vanilla extract

1 tablespoon coconut oil

2 medjool dates, pitted

1 cup fresh blueberries

Combine the almond flour, tapioca flour, coconut flour, baking powder, salt, eggs, oat milk, and vanilla extract in a large bowl and whisk until it becomes a smooth batter.

Heat the coconut oil in a nonstick pan. When the pan is hot, ladle in 2 tablespoons of batter, carefully forming a circular shape. If there is extra space, you can cook more pancakes at once, leaving ½ inch between pancakes. Let them cook on one side for 2 minutes or until the edges and bottom are golden brown. Flip and do the same with the other side.

Put the pitted dates in a small saucepan and cover with water. Bring to a boil and reduce until it has a consistency slightly looser than honey. Add the blueberries and ¼ cup water. As the water comes back to a boil, mash the blueberries down and reduce the liquid until it has a syrupy consistency.

Enjoy the pancakes with 1 tablespoon of the blueberry syrup.

Overnight Oats and Chia Bowl

I like making these in glass jars so I can just pick one up in the morning and eat it whenever I want. When I eat overnight oats at home, I enjoy them with some fried eggs and a hot cup of coffee.

SERVES 2

1 cup rolled oats

2 tablespoons chia seeds

1 teaspoon ground cinnamon

¼ cup freeze-dried fruit of your choice

2 cups unsweetened oat or almond milk

¼ cup fresh berries

¼ cup granola

Prepare this meal at least 6 hours before consuming. Combine the rolled oats, chia seeds, cinnamon, freeze-dried fruit, and unsweetened milk of your choice. Mix thoroughly. Cover the container and refrigerate for at least 6 hours.

When you're ready to consume it, place about 1 cup of the overnight oat mixture in a bowl, loosening it up with more oat or almond milk if you'd like. Top with some fresh berries, granola, and another dash of cinnamon.

Kale Chips

This is an easy recipe for when you want to have that bag-of-chips feeling without the guilt that may come with it when you know what's in most chips you can buy at the grocery store, LOL.

1 bunch kale, stemmed

2 tablespoons sunflower or coconut oil

½ teaspoon cayenne pepper

½ teaspoon ground garlic powder

½ teaspoon sea salt

Preheat the oven to 300°F. Make sure to remove all the woody stems of the kale and cut the leaves into 1-inch pieces. Put the kale in a large bowl and add the other ingredients. Massage the kale thoroughly so it is evenly coated.

Line a baking sheet with foil and lay the kale out evenly. Place the baking sheet in the oven and bake for about 10 minutes. Turn the kale over so the other side can bake for an additional 5 minutes, or until edges are golden brown.

Cool the kale chips and enjoy!

Egg-Salad-Stuffed Celery

This is a great snack for having at work or taking with you on trips. Just buy a little cooler and glass containers to take it with you.

4 hard-boiled eggs, peeled

¼ cup Greek yogurt

1 tablespoon Dijon mustard

2 tablespoons white vinegar

5 sprigs fresh dill, picked and roughly chopped

Sea salt and cracked black pepper to taste

1 head celery, cut into 3-inch logs

Put the hard-boiled eggs in a bowl. Gently break them into quarters with a fork and then add the yogurt, mustard, vinegar, and dill. Mix all the ingredients as you continue to break apart the eggs. Season with salt and pepper to taste.

Assemble by putting ½ tablespoon egg salad on each log of celery.

Hummus

Who doesn't like hummus?! This recipe goes really well with my sweet potatoes and some fish if you want to go from snack to full meal.

1 can chickpeas, drained

2 cloves fresh garlic, grated

3 lemons, juiced

¼ cup tahini

½ teaspoon paprika

Ice water, as needed

1 tablespoon olive oil

Sea salt to taste

Your choice of raw vegetables, cut into sticks

Cover the chickpeas with water in a pot. Bring to a boil, and boil for about 15 minutes. Remove from the heat, allow to cool, and remove any skins that may still be on the chickpeas.

Put the cooked chickpeas in a food processor with the garlic and process for about 20 seconds. Add lemon juice and process until it looks like a loose paste. Add tahini and paprika and continue to process. If it gets too thick, slowly drizzle in ice water, one tablespoon at a time. When you're happy with the consistency, drizzle in olive oil and salt to taste.

Enjoy with your favorite vegetables. I like raw carrot sticks, celery sticks, and radishes.

Guacamole with Sweet Potato Chips

I love aguacates (avocados)! This snack is a weekend favorite and best enjoyed with friends, so start planning that brunch-at-home party and impress yo' friends with your newfound cooking skills!

1 sweet potato

2 tablespoons sunflower or coconut oil

Cayenne pepper to taste

1 teaspoon sea salt

1 ripe avocado

½ small red onion, diced

¼ bunch cilantro, finely chopped

½ lime, juiced

Preheat the oven to 400°F. Using a sharp mandoline slicer, slice the sweet potato as thin as possible so the chips can get nice and crispy. Put the slices in a large bowl and mix with the oil, cayenne pepper, and salt, coating the slices evenly.

Spread the sweet potato slices on a baking sheet lined with parchment paper. Make sure there is at least one centimeter of space between adjacent chips.

Place the baking sheet in the oven and bake for about 10 minutes. When the chips begin to look golden brown, turn them over and bake for another 10 minutes. Remove from the oven and let the chips cool on a cooling rack so they stay crispy.

Meanwhile, cut the avocado in half, remove the pit, and scoop out the pulp into a bowl. Add the onion and cilantro. Mix gently—you don't want to overwork the avocado because it can become gummy. Add the lime juice and a pinch of salt to taste. Mash the guacamole around until all the ingredients are fully incorporated and you are happy with the consistency.

There is *always* room for dessert! Well, for you it is every 10 days, but you get it. Let's make some delicious goodness, shall we?

Dark Chocolate Nutty Bark

For when you're craving some chocolate, like I do once a month. ;)

1 pound 70% dark chocolate

½ cup roasted almonds, roughly chopped

½ cup roasted walnuts, roughly chopped

¼ cup puffed quinoa (optional, for texture)

¼ cup roasted sunflower seeds

Use a knife to chop the chocolate into small, thin pieces and place in a stainless-steel bowl. Fill a small saucepot halfway with water and bring to a boil. Reduce the boil to a simmer. Let the bowl of chocolate rest on the rim of the saucepot, over the boiling water. Stir the chocolate pieces until they are completely melted.

Remove the bowl of melted chocolate from the heat. Evenly distribute the almonds, walnuts, quinoa, and sunflower seeds in the bowl of chocolate. Stir so everything is evenly mixed into the melted chocolate.

Spread the mixture onto a baking sheet lined with parchment paper. Let it cool in the refrigerator to harden, then break it up into pieces.

Blueberry Banana Pops

These are a great summer brunch option and something you can make for your kids, your sister's kids, the neighborhood kids—you get the point!

MAKES 6 TO 8 POPS

3 cups fresh blueberries

2 large bananas, ripe

½ cup Greek yogurt

1 cup unsweetened oat milk

1 teaspoon vanilla extract

½ teaspoon ground cinnamon

Throw all the ingredients into a blender and blend until completely smooth. Add more oat milk if needed.

Pour the blueberry banana mixture into frozen treat molds and place them in the freezer. They will take at least 3 hours to become completely frozen.

Flourless Chocolate Cake

This has been one of my favorites since basically forever—I love me a melty chocolate cake right after dinner. I highly recommend you have this with some of your fave ice cream for that cheat you're earning thanks to your hard work. Enjoy!

SERVES 2

4 medjool dates, pitted

200 grams 70% dark chocolate (or 64% if you want it sweeter)

½ cup coconut oil

¼ cup cocoa powder

1 teaspoon vanilla extract

½ teaspoon sea salt

3 eggs

Preheat the oven to 375°F. Use a little bit of coconut oil to grease the inside of an 8-inch springform cake pan.

Put the pitted dates in a small saucepan and cover with water. Bring to a boil and reduce until it is a thick consistency, like honey. Make sure it is completely cool before moving on.

Use a knife to chop the chocolate into small, thin pieces. Put the chocolate and coconut oil in a stainless-steel bowl. Fill a small saucepot halfway with water and bring to a boil. Reduce the boil to a simmer. Let the bowl of chocolate rest on the rim of the saucepot, over the boiling water. Stir the chocolate pieces and coconut oil until everything is completely melted.

In a stand mixer, combine the melted chocolate, medjool date honey, cocoa powder, vanilla extract, and salt and begin to whisk slowly. Once everything is combined, speed up the mixer and add the three eggs until the batter is smooth.

Transfer the batter to the springform pan and bake for about 20 minutes or until the cake is firm and a cake tester or toothpick inserted into the center comes out clean. Cool before you enjoy it! This cake freezes well, so you can enjoy it for up to one month.

Oatmeal Almond Cookies

Fresh, warm cookies always make me feel like a kid again. It's time you bring some of that nostalgia into your life. I enjoy mine with some cold almond milk.

SERVES 4

4 medjool dates, pitted

2 cups rolled oats

1 cup almond flour

¼ cup unsweetened coconut flakes

½ cup toasted almonds

1 tablespoon cinnamon

⅓ cup coconut oil, melted

1 teaspoon vanilla extract

1 teaspoon sea salt

Preheat the oven to 350°F and line a baking sheet with parchment paper.

Put the pitted dates in a small saucepan and cover with water. Bring to a boil and reduce until it is a thick consistency, like honey. Make sure it is completely cool before moving on.

Mix together the oats, almond flour, coconut flakes, almonds, and cinnamon. In a separate bowl, mix together the date honey, coconut oil, vanilla extract, and salt. Slowly stir the coconut oil mixture into the almond flour mixture. When everything is mixed together, form two-inch balls and place them on the baking sheet with at least one inch of space between balls.

Place the baking sheet in the oven and bake for 20 minutes, or until the cookies are golden brown. Remove from the oven and allow to cool before you enjoy!

Banana Chocolate Bread

Where do I begin with this guy?! I make this for my kid's school events and end up eating "some" (more like half) of it every time. This can easily be turned into the base for a delicious cake as well.

SERVES 4

1 tablespoon sunflower or coconut oil

2½ cups almond flour

2 teaspoons baking powder

½ teaspoon sea salt

4 small bananas, mashed

3 eggs

1 teaspoon pure vanilla extract

¼ cup dark chocolate chips

Preheat the oven to 350°F and use a little bit of the oil to grease the inside of a loaf pan. You can also line the bottom of the loaf pan with parchment paper if you wish.

In a stand mixer, combine the almond flour, baking powder, and salt. Mix well.

Continue mixing slowly as you add the mashed bananas. Once they are fully mixed in, add the eggs, one by one. Then add the oil and vanilla extract. Using a spatula, fold in the chocolate chips.

Pour the batter into the loaf pan and bake for about 30 minutes. Check to see if it is done by inserting a cake tester or toothpick in the middle. If the tester does not come out clean, return the pan to the oven and bake for another 5 to 10 minutes. Remove from the oven when the cake tester comes out clean.

Let the bread cool so it can hold its shape when removed from the pan.

Gluten-Free Sweet Potato Pie

Have it for Thanksgiving, have it during Christmas, have it on a random Friday night, LOL. I like to add some whipped cream or ice cream on mine, just sayin'!

SERVES 4

For the crust

1 cup rolled oats

1 cup raw almonds

½ cup raw walnuts

4 medjool dates, pitted and chopped

2 teaspoons ground cinnamon

1 teaspoon sea salt

¼ cup coconut oil, melted

For the filling

2 medium sweet potatoes

2 medjool dates, pitted

2 eggs

½ cup unsweetened almond milk

1 teaspoon ground cinnamon

1 teaspoon ground ginger

1 teaspoon pure vanilla extract

2 teaspoons lemon juice

1 teaspoon sea salt

Preheat the oven to 400°F and grease the inside of a 9-inch pie pan with a little bit of coconut oil.

For the pie crust, put the oats, almonds, walnuts, chopped dates, cinnamon, and salt in a food processor and process until you get an even, crumbly texture. Then slowly add the melted coconut oil until it becomes almost like a paste.

Press the pie crust mixture evenly into the pan and place in the refrigerator for 20 minutes so the crust can set.

Bake the sweet potatoes in the preheated oven for 40 minutes or until tender when poked with a fork. When ready, remove them from the oven and allow them to cool. Peel the skins and discard.

Put the remaining pitted dates in a small saucepan and cover with water. Bring to a boil and reduce until it is a thick consistency, like honey. Make sure it is completely cool before moving on.

In a blender, combine the cooked sweet potatoes, date honey, eggs, almond milk, cinnamon, ginger, vanilla extract, lemon juice, and salt. Mix until the pie filling is smooth and creamy. Pour it evenly into the pie shell.

Place the pie into the oven and bake for 15 minutes. Lower the temperature to 325°F and continue to bake for another 30 minutes, or until the edges are firm and the middle has a very slight jiggle. Remove from the oven and let it rest for at least 1 hour. The residual heat will continue to cook the pie even when it is out of the oven. Enjoy the pie at room temperature or place it in the refrigerator to enjoy it cold.

Exercise Database

Adductor Machine

BODY PART: Legs
EQUIPMENT: Adductor machine

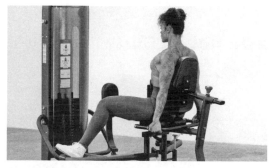

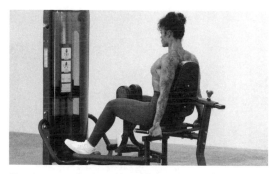

To target your adductors, be sure to squeeze your back muscles and tuck your butt in as you squeeze your inner thighs.

Push your knees in with control and power, then slowly open them back up before repeating.

Air Squat

BODY PART: Legs
EQUIPMENT: Bodyweight

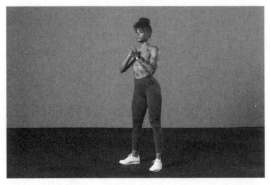

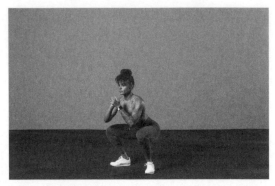

Keep your chest up nice and high with your weight in your heels.

Get a bit lower than 90 degrees and really push yourself off the ground to work that booty, moving fluidly.

Alternating Biceps Dumbbell Curl

BODY PART: Biceps
EQUIPMENT: Dumbbells

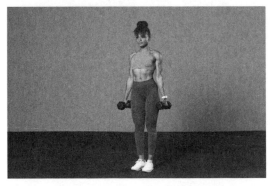

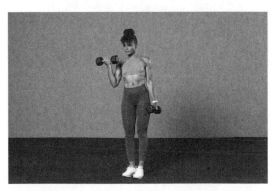

Engage your core and sit into your hips so you don't twist your torso.

Make sure you curl each arm up with control; avoid swinging or moving your chest forward and backward.

Alternating Knee to Elbow

BODY PART: Abs
EQUIPMENT: Bodyweight

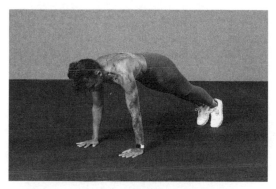

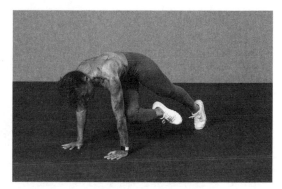

Get into the plank position. Round your upper back and tuck the butt in. Now bring your right knee to your left elbow, and vice versa.

Exhale as you bring your knee to elbow and inhale as it moves back.

Arnold Press

BODY PART: Shoulders
EQUIPMENT: Dumbbells

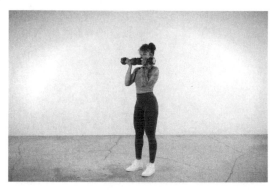

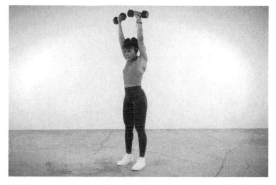

Rotate and raise the dumbbells at the same time; this will keep the tension in your shoulders as you're working.

Make sure not to let the dumbbells fall past your chin on the way down.

Assisted Dip

BODY PART: Triceps
EQUIPMENT: Dip stand with band

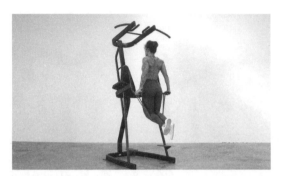 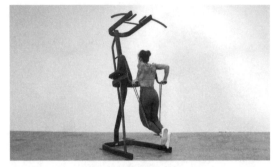

Although these are assisted, you're still going to get great activation of key muscles in your chest, shoulders, and triceps. (If you find you need more support than the band, check to see if your gym has an assisted dip machine.)

Keep your elbows pointed back; do not flare them out to the sides. Lower down to 90 degrees in the elbows.

Banded Diagonal-Forward Crab Walk

BODY PART: Legs
EQUIPMENT: Band

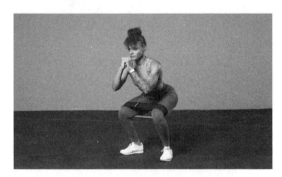 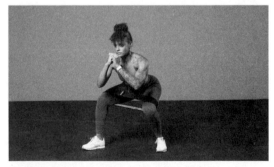

Place a hip band right above your knees and get into a chair position (lower part of the squat). Keep your chest out and back straight.

Now take a step to the side and forward, and follow with your other foot, continuing this pattern until you finish the prescribed number of reps.

Banded Hamstring Curl

BODY PART: Legs
EQUIPMENT: Band, bench

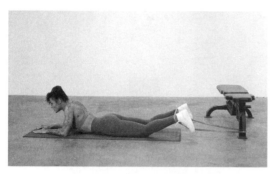

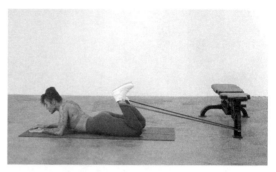

Make sure you start with enough tension in your resistance band.

Move your feet down slowly until you feel the burn before coming back up.

Banded Step-Out

BODY PART: Legs
EQUIPMENT: Band

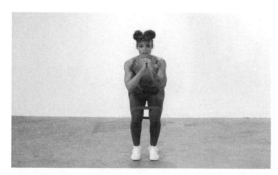

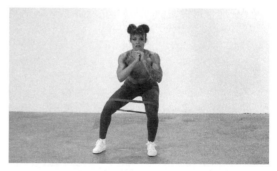

Bend your legs and sit back into a low squat.

Tap out with each leg, keeping your knee in line with your toes. Keep a tight posture.

Banded Straight-Arm Pull-Down

BODY PART: Back
EQUIPMENT: Band, barbell stand

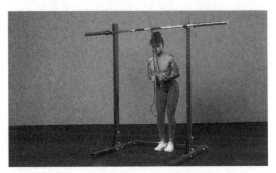 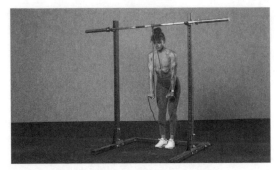

Keep your dominant foot slightly forward; this is where most of your weight will be. Start with the band at the same level as your diaphragm.

Keep your chest up to prevent your shoulders from caving in. Exhale and pull down; control the movement on the way up and keep your reps smooth.

Barbell Drag Curl

BODY PART: Biceps
EQUIPMENT: Barbell

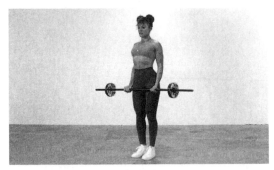 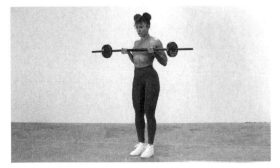

Keep the bar close to your body as you drag it up in a straight line vertically. Your elbows should be right by your sides as you drag.

Most important: Keep your shoulders back and chest forward.

Barbell Flat Chest Press

BODY PART: Chest
EQUIPMENT: Barbell, bench

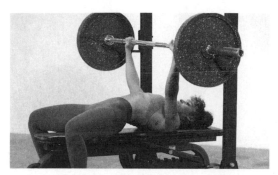

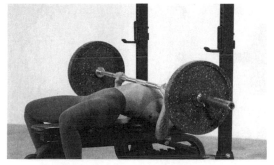

Press your back flat into the bench and set feet flat on the ground. Make sure the bar is under eye level. For all presses, you want your feet planted on the floor, butt firmly on the bench, shoulder blades retracted, and chest out, which will slightly arch your lower back (bridging).

Lower the bar down slowly to your diaphragm and then back up. Keep your chest out, squeeze your pecs, and keep your reps smooth.

Barbell Incline Chest Press

BODY PART: Chest
EQUIPMENT: Barbell, incline bench

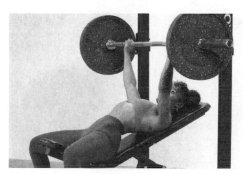

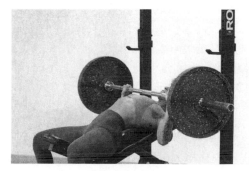

Focus on your form. Your chest needs to be up, with your shoulders back.

Concentrate and really push yourself on this one, breathing through the move.

Barbell Preacher Curl

BODY PART: Biceps
EQUIPMENT: Barbell, incline bench

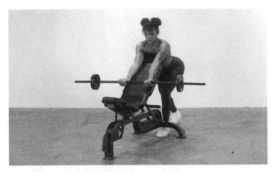 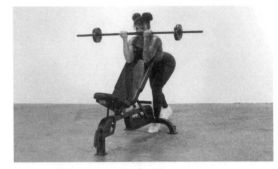

This will feel harder than a normal curl. Make sure your wrists are straight and you are moving through the full range of motion.

Barbell Row (Supinated Grip)

BODY PART: Back
EQUIPMENT: Barbell

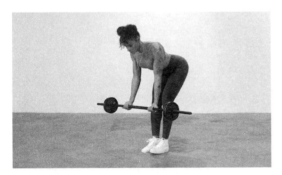 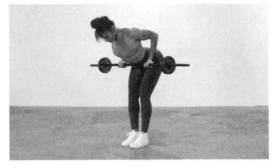

Sit into your hips and engage your core. Keep your chest forward and shoulder blades back as you pull the bar toward your ribs. Think about squeezing a pencil between your shoulder blades.

Hold for 1 second at the top before lowering back down. "Supinated" means holding the bar from underneath.

Bent-Over Dumbbell Row

BODY PART: Back
EQUIPMENT: Dumbbells

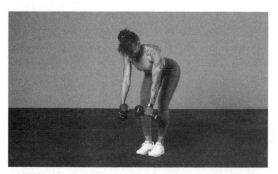 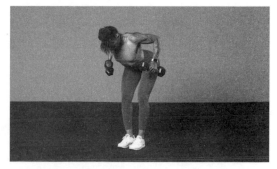

Start in a standing position and slowly bend your knees and then upper body until you're at about a 60-degree angle.

Drive your elbows back, squeeze your shoulder blades, and bring the dumbbells down to the initial position in a controlled way.

Bent-Over Rear Delt Barbell Row

BODY PART: Shoulders
EQUIPMENT: Barbell

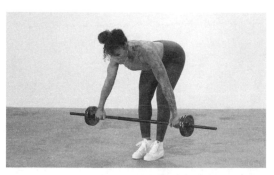 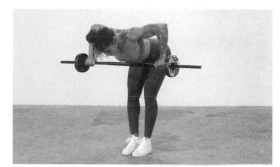

The wide grip here will really target your upper back and rear delts.

Bend your knees slightly and bring your chest down toward the floor. Lead with your elbows toward the ceiling and keep your core tight.

Bent-Over Smith Machine Row (Supinated Grip)

BODY PART: Back
EQUIPMENT: Smith machine

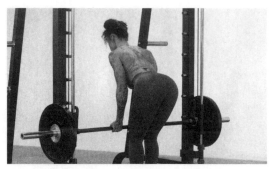

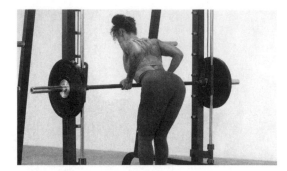

Focus on pulling the bar toward your ribs while keeping your core engaged the entire time; you don't want to move from your initial position.

Keep a long, straight back.

Biceps Barbell Curl

BODY PART: Biceps
EQUIPMENT: Barbell

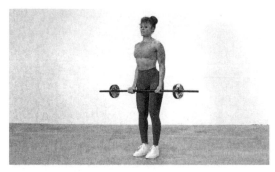

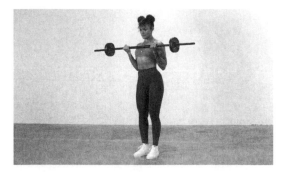

This exercise really isolates the biceps. Keep your elbows to your side and move with control.

Bring the bar up to chin level before going back down.

Biceps E-Z Bar Curl

BODY PART: Biceps
EQUIPMENT: E-Z bar

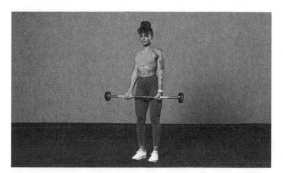

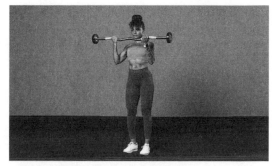

As with the barbell, the goal is to isolate the biceps, except that now we give them a little extra engagement.

Make sure to fully engage your biceps on the way up. Control the E-Z bar on the way down, squeezing your triceps. At the bottom of each rep, roll right into the next one.

Biceps Rope Curl

BODY PART: Biceps
EQUIPMENT: Cable machine

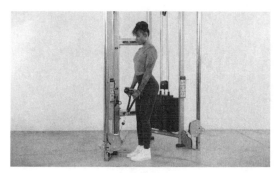

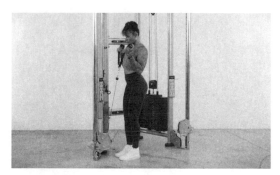

Make sure to take one step away from the cable machine before beginning your curls. Your knees should be slightly bent as you sit into your hips with your chest up.

Keep your elbows close to your obliques as you pull up.

Biceps Straight-Bar Curl

BODY PART: Biceps
EQUIPMENT: Cable machine

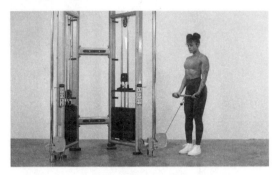

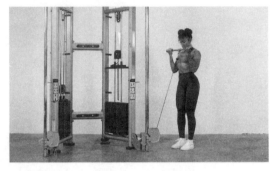

Keep your elbows tucked, chest up, and your core super tight.

Most important: Be sure to keep your wrists straight.

Bicycle Sprint

BODY PART: Full body (cardio)
EQUIPMENT: Stationary bicycle

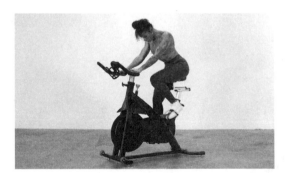

Alternate sprints with riding at a normal pace for the designated amount of time.

Push yourself with this exercise—I want you to give it everything you've got. Cardio is about keeping your heart healthy and burning fat!

Bulgarian Split Squat

BODY PART: Legs
EQUIPMENT: Dumbbells, bench

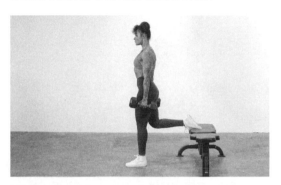 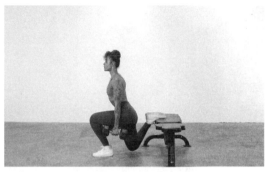

We're working one leg at a time here, which means you will really feel this in your quads. Get as low as you can while keeping your chest high.

It's okay if your front knee goes slightly past your toe; just give yourself enough space between the bench and your front foot.

Cable Chest Fly

BODY PART: Chest
EQUIPMENT: Cable machine

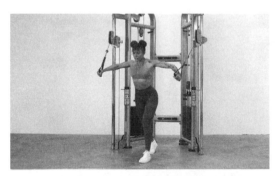 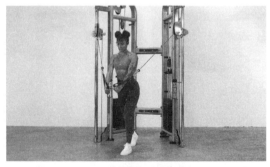

Stand with your legs staggered and your knees slightly flexed for a good base. Make sure to keep a steady bend in the elbows.

Squeeze your chest tight and hold for a brief pause before opening back up.

Cable Glute Kick-Back

BODY PART: Legs
EQUIPMENT: Cable machine

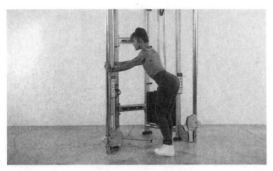

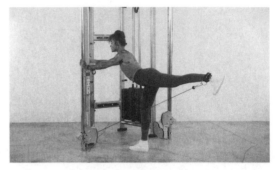

Keep a slight bend in both knees. Flex the foot on your working leg and kick up in a swift motion to get the most out of the movement.

This is a great exercise for the booty.

Cable Row

BODY PART: Back
EQUIPMENT: Cable machine

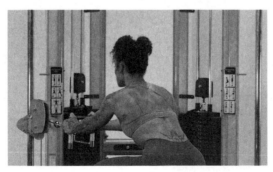

Lean forward as much as you can to start this move. When you pull back, lead with your elbows and let the bar touch your belly.

Lean back slightly at the end and squeeze your shoulder blades, holding for a brief second before lowering back down. You can also use a row machine for this exercise.

Chest Dip (Assisted)

BODY PART: Chest
EQUIPMENT: Dip stand with band

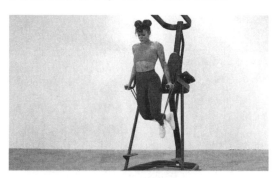 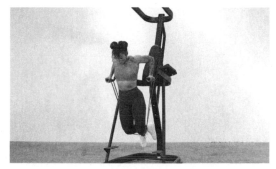

Focus on your form and take advantage of the band on this one. (If you find you need more support than the band, check to see if your gym has an assisted dip machine.)

Keep your chin tucked the entire time as you move down to a 90-degree bend in the elbow with control.

Crab Walk (Bodyweight)

BODY PART: Legs
EQUIPMENT: Bodyweight

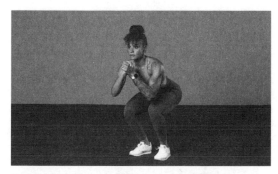 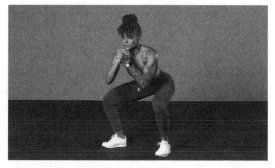

Stay in a deep squat the entire time with this exercise. Keep your core super tight and chest lifted. Step sideways with one leg, then the other leg follows in the same direction. Think walking sideways like a crab.

You can keep your arms forward to help with balance.

Dead Lift

BODY PART: Legs
EQUIPMENT: Barbell

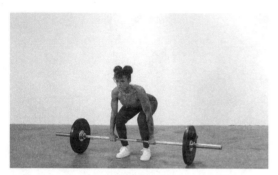

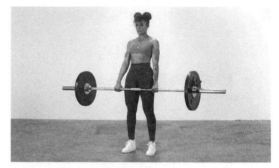

This is one of the best moves for building muscle in the lower body. Start by pushing your hips back and keep the bar close to your legs during the entire movement.

Keep your core engaged and make sure your chest is high and shoulders are back. Push off your feet and drive your hips forward to stand up. Be sure to control the movement on the way down into the next rep.

Decline Sit-Up

BODY PART: Abs
EQUIPMENT: Decline bench

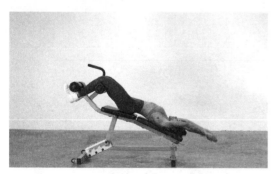

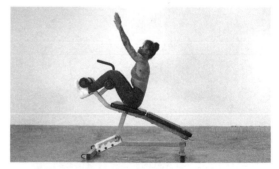

Keep your chest up and push your shoulders back throughout this exercise. Look up at the ceiling to really engage your core.

Move slowly on the way down, taking 2 to 3 seconds to really engage your abs all the way through this move.

Dip (Bodyweight)

BODY PART: Triceps
EQUIPMENT: Dip stand

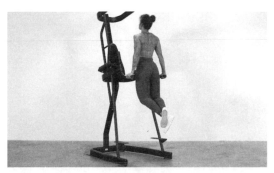 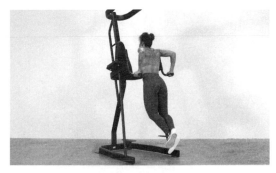

Start at the top of the movement, and lower only to a 90-degree bend in the elbows. Look straight ahead the entire time.

This is a tough move, so keep using a band, machine, or bench for assistance if needed.

Drop Squat (Banded)

BODY PART: Legs
EQUIPMENT: Bodyweight, band

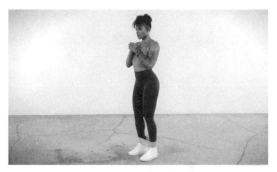 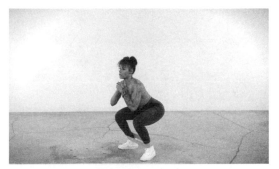

I want you to go for a deep squat each time. Keep your core super tight and chest lifted.

Start with feet hip-width apart, and shift quickly into a wide stance as you drop—you're basically doing a tiny jump. You can keep your arms forward to help balance.

Dumbbell Flat Chest Press

BODY PART: Chest
EQUIPMENT: Dumbbells, bench

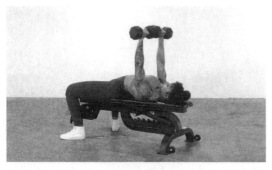

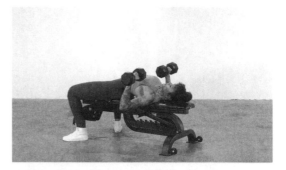

Lower the weights down till they hit your chest right under your armpits.

Press straight up, keeping your shoulders down and away from your ears.

Dumbbell Incline Biceps Curl

BODY PART: Biceps
EQUIPMENT: Dumbbells, incline bench

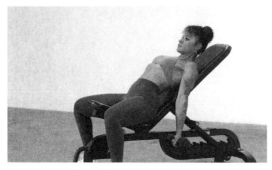

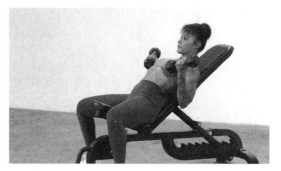

We're really isolating your biceps here. It's important to move with control and breathe through the move.

Lock your upper arms into place while keeping your wrists straight.

Dumbbell Incline Chest Press

BODY PART: Chest
EQUIPMENT: Dumbbells, incline bench

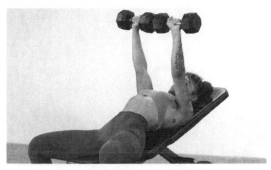

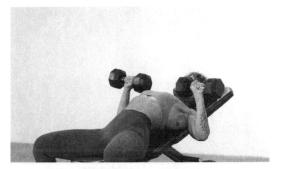

We're using an incline bench with this exercise to activate more muscle fibers within your chest.

Keep your chest high, shoulders back, and really engage your chest at the top of the movement.

Dumbbell Static Lunge

BODY PART: Legs
EQUIPMENT: Dumbbells

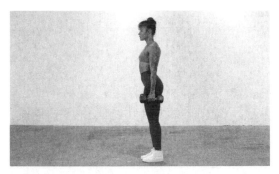

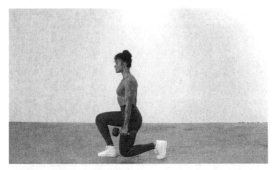

Move slowly forward, taking two seconds on the way down, then pausing briefly at the bottom. You want your body to move up and down in a straight line.

Focus on getting low without your rear knee hitting the ground. Your front knee should be aligned with your toes.

Dumbbell Stiff-Leg Dead Lift

BODY PART: Legs
EQUIPMENT: Dumbbells

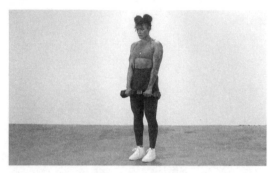 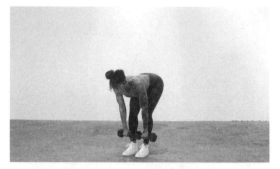

We're working on your hamstrings and underbutt with this one. Keep a slight bend in your knees as you move down with the dumbbells.

Keep your chest and shoulders engaged and squeeze your butt hard at the top.

E-Z Bar Skull Crusher on Bench

BODY PART: Triceps
EQUIPMENT: E-Z bar, bench

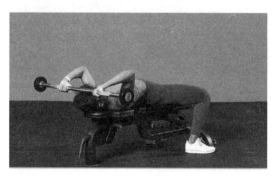 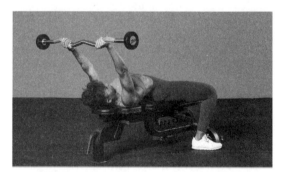

Keep your upper arms and elbows locked in. Only your forearms should move in this one.

Face Pull

BODY PART: Back
EQUIPMENT: Cable machine

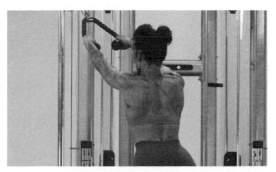

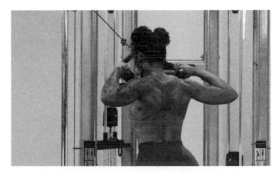

We're working on your rear delts here (the back part of your shoulder).

You should be pulling with your hands and leading with your elbows. Keep those elbows high to hit the right area.

Foam Rolling

BODY PART: Full body (recovery)
EQUIPMENT: Foam roller

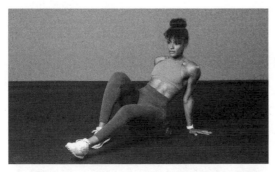

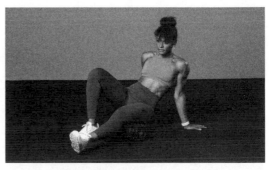

It's easier than you think! Start high up on your back, roll forward, then back a bit more down toward your lower back.

Repeat the same process, starting with your upper body and ending with your quads, hamstrings, and calves.

Front Raise

BODY PART: Shoulders
EQUIPMENT: Dumbbells

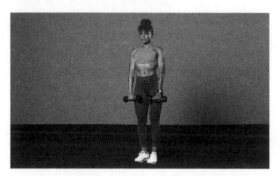

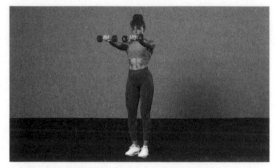

Keep your core engaged and avoid overarching your back.

Exhale and lift the dumbbells right in front of you to about chin level. Squeeze your shoulders at the top and move the weights back down with control.

Front Squat

BODY PART: Legs
EQUIPMENT: Barbell

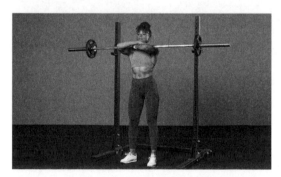

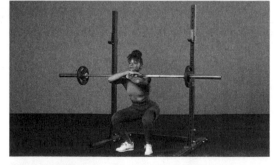

Keep your feet about hip-width apart, chest up, and hold the barbell right above your chest while keeping the elbows parallel with the floor.

Control the movement on the way down, then exhale and go up, focusing on your quads and hips. Make sure to come down to just past parallel with the floor.

Goblet Squat

BODY PART: Legs
EQUIPMENT: Dumbbells

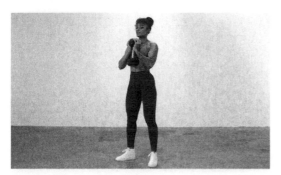

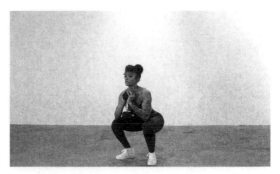

Start with your feet slightly wider than hip-width apart. Use a heavy or challenging weight for this one. Go deep into your squat, slightly past 90 degrees, while keeping your chest nice and high.

Push through your heels to stand back up, moving in a fluid motion through this exercise.

Good Morning

BODY PART: Legs
EQUIPMENT: Barbell

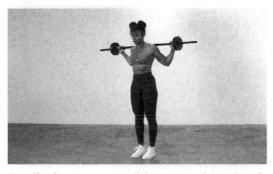

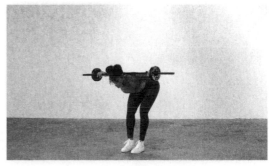

Really focus on pushing your hips back first, before lowering your chest.

Keep your knees slightly bent to protect your lower back.

Hamstring Curl (Cable)

BODY PART: Legs
EQUIPMENT: Cable machine

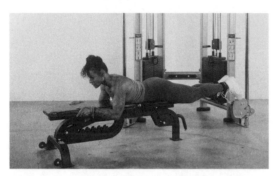

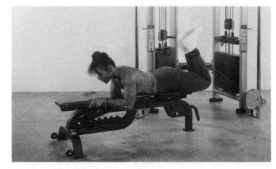

The key to this exercise is to not let your knees drop lower than the bench.

Flex your feet and kick your heels up to your booty. Keep your spine neutral by looking forward the entire time.

Hamstring Curl Machine

BODY PART: Legs
EQUIPMENT: Hamstring curl machine

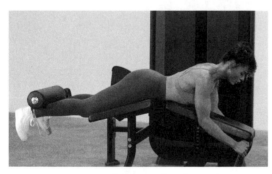

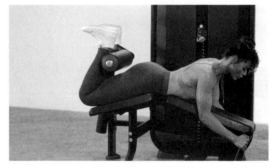

Keep your hips flat on the bench. Your chest should be up and your shoulders back.

These are going to hurt, but they are so worth it!

Hamstring Extension Machine

BODY PART: Legs
EQUIPMENT: Hamstring extension machine

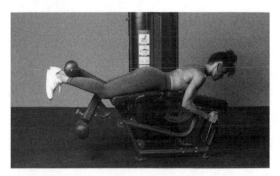 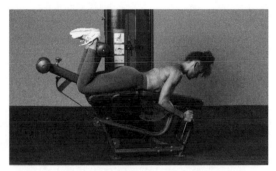

This machine isolates your hamstrings and can be used to develop your engagement in those muscles.

Make sure to keep your back and neck aligned. Exhale when you lift and control the weight on your way down before going back up.

Hanging Leg Lift

BODY PART: Abs
EQUIPMENT: Rack

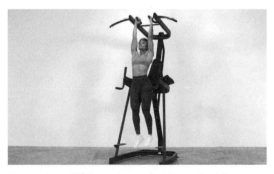 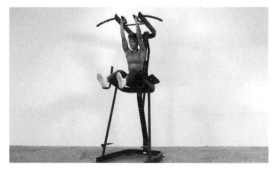

Focus on lifting your feet up to the level of your hips.

To avoid swinging, try locking in your chest and your lats. Push your chest forward as you move your legs up.

High Knees

BODY PART: Full body (cardio)
EQUIPMENT: Bodyweight

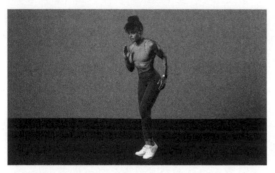

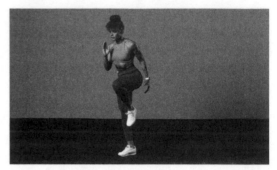

This looks like a leg exercise, but it's really a killer core movement!

Start in the standing position and bring one knee to hip level, then switch legs with power and control while switching your arms along with them.

Hip Thrust (Barbell, Banded)

BODY PART: Legs
EQUIPMENT: Barbell, band, bench

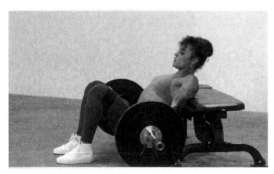

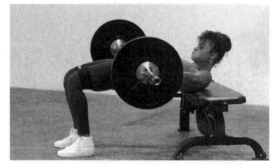

Start by placing the edge of the bench right below your shoulder blades, place your feet wider than hip-width apart, and align your head with your back.

Thrust the bar all the way up until you have a flat line from your knees to shoulders. Look straight ahead the entire time while keeping your chin tucked.

Hip Thrust (Bodyweight, Banded)

BODY PART: Legs
EQUIPMENT: Band

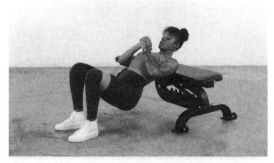 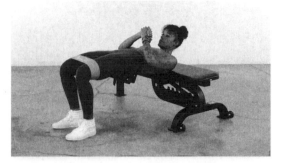

Start by placing the edge of the bench right below your shoulder blades, place your feet wider than hip-width apart, and align your head with your back.

Tuck your chin in and keep your eyes forward. Move only your hips as you perform a scooping motion on the way up.

Hip Thrust (Smith Machine)

BODY PART: Legs
EQUIPMENT: Smith machine

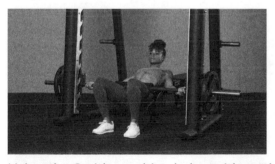 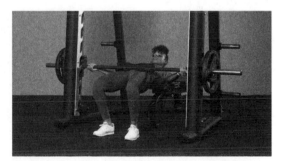

Using the Smith machine helps with setting up and building your way to barbell thrusts!

Set the bar aligned with your hips, keep your eyes looking forward, and set your shoulder blades right above the edge of the bench. Exhale on the work and control the movement on the way down.

Hip-Up (Banded)

BODY PART: Legs
EQUIPMENT: Band

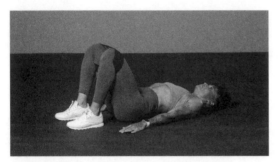

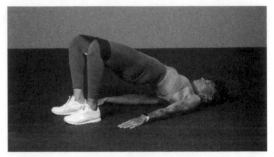

Place either your feet on the floor or your midfoot on the bench edge, and drive your hips up while keeping your shoulder blades flat on the floor. Exhale on the way up and squeeze your core.

Look straight ahead the entire time while keeping your chin tucked.

Hot Yoga

BODY PART: Full body (recovery)
EQUIPMENT: N/A

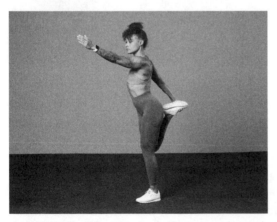

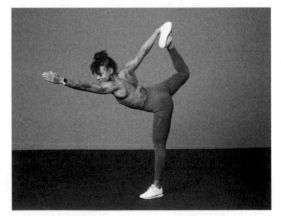

Any 45- to 60-minute hot yoga class that you like will be perfect; just find one you enjoy since the heat and stretching of the muscles is what you need.

In-and-Out Abs

BODY PART: Abs
EQUIPMENT: Bodyweight

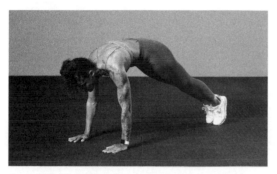 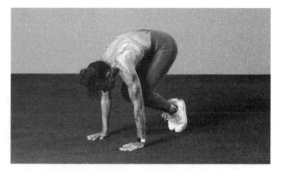

Start in the plank position. Squeeze your shoulder blades together, tuck your butt in, and bring your feet together.

Drive your knees and feet forward toward your chest, land softly, and jump right back. Keep your reps nice and smooth.

Incline Leg Lift

BODY PART: Abs
EQUIPMENT: Incline bench

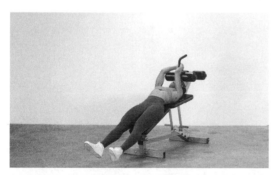 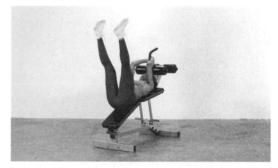

This one is going to burn. Focus on using your abs to lift your legs by pushing your back into the bench really hard. Make sure to look up at the ceiling.

Incline Smith Machine Press

BODY PART: Chest
EQUIPMENT: Smith machine

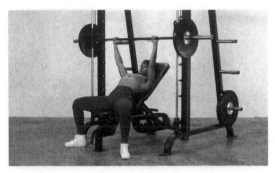 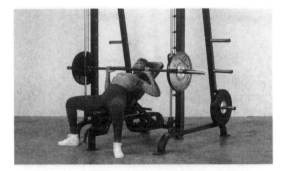

Same as the Smith machine flat chest press, just at an angle. Sit with your butt tucked in, abs contracted, and chest out. Your feet need to be planted flat in front of you.

Keep your chest out and squeeze your pecs as you press upward. Control the movement on the way back, and keep your reps smooth.

Jump Rope

BODY PART: Full body (cardio)
EQUIPMENT: Jump rope

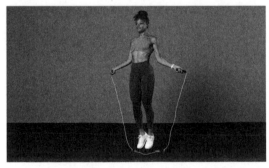 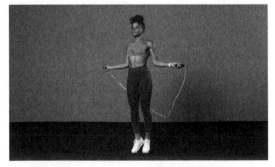

Set the rope length to just about past your hips.

As you jump, your goal is to land smoothly and concentrate on connecting your breathing to the tempo of the rope. Enjoy!

Jumping Jack

BODY PART: Full body (cardio)
EQUIPMENT: Bodyweight

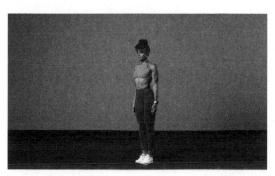 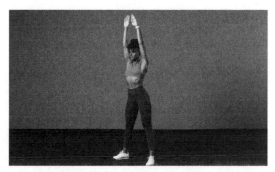

Keep your eyes looking straight ahead. Your arms and legs move together and open up. Make sure to keep your shoulder blades contracted and your chest out the entire time—don't just swing your arms.

Your goal is to control the movement and land smoothly and almost silently.

KB Dead Lift to Squat

BODY PART: Legs
EQUIPMENT: Kettlebell

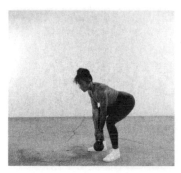 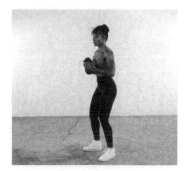 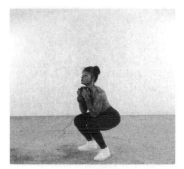

As you move up from the dead lift position, start pulling the weight with your hands. Use your momentum to switch the weight to your hands and drop into a squat. Make sure to hold the KB right on your chest with your arms in and elbows pointing straight down as you switch from the dead lift into the squat position.

KB Pulsating Squat

BODY PART: Legs
EQUIPMENT: Kettlebell

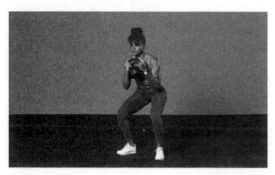 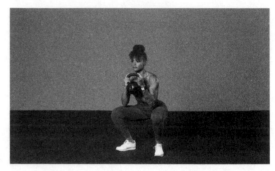

Assume a squat position, and hold KB in front of you. Get low and keep your shoulders away from your ears. Sit low into your squat and pulse up and down no more than an inch.

KB Pulsating Sumo

BODY PART: Legs
EQUIPMENT: Kettlebell

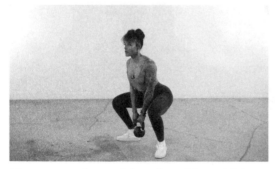 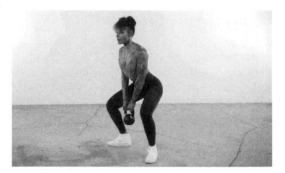

Keep your feet wider than hip-width apart and your chest up. Get low and keep your shoulders away from your ears. Sit low into your squat and pulse up and down no more than an inch, with the KB between your legs.

KB Single-Arm Row

BODY PART: Back
EQUIPMENT: Kettlebell

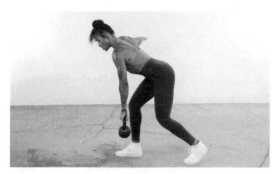 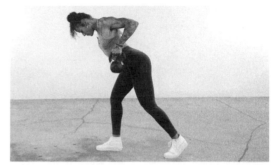

Focus on keeping your chest up and your shoulders back. Lead with your elbow as you draw the weight up.

KB Single-Leg Lunge

BODY PART: Legs
EQUIPMENT: Kettlebell

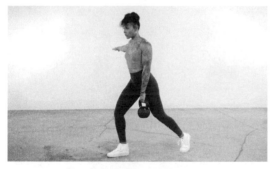 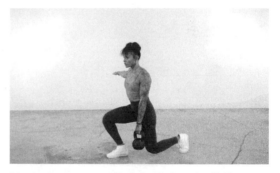

Bring your rear leg to a 90-degree angle on your way down. It's okay if your front knee tracks out past your toe.

Keep your core tight and put all the weight into your front heel. Be sure to hold the weight perpendicular to your body so that your palm faces your leg.

KB Swing

BODY PART: Legs
EQUIPMENT: Kettlebell

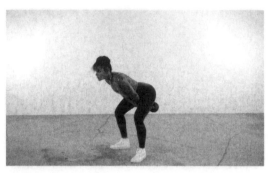

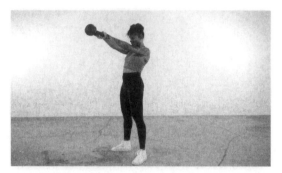

Relax your hands and arms. You want the kettlebell to fall between your knees by hinging your hips back.

Remember to push from your hips, bringing the kettlebell to eye level.

Kick-Back (Bodyweight)

BODY PART: Legs
EQUIPMENT: Bodyweight

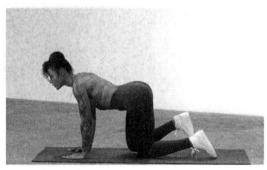

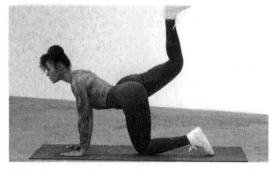

Focus on leading with your heel, kicking the bottom of your foot up at the ceiling.

This is a really great accessory exercise to support your bigger movement patterns such as squats and dead lifts. These should be done at a dynamic pace so you feel the burn, but always with control!

Kneeling Rope Crunch

BODY PART: Abs
EQUIPMENT: Cable machine

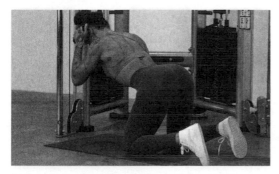

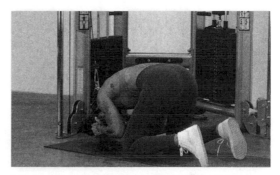

Use your core the entire time. Your thumbs should be on your temples. Arch hard and crunch hard.

It's important that your neck stay in line with your spine here to avoid injury.

Lat Pull-Down (Supinated Narrow Grip)

BODY PART: Back
EQUIPMENT: Lat pull-down machine

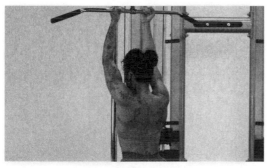

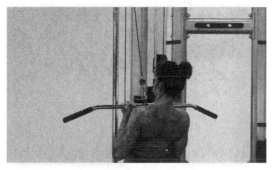

This is going to really work your mid-back. Keep your chest up and core engaged. Make sure to hold the bar with your palms facing you.

As you pull the bar down, lead with your elbows and lean back slightly. Keep your shoulders away from your ears.

Lat Pull-Down (Wide Grip)

BODY PART: Back
EQUIPMENT: Lat pull-down machine

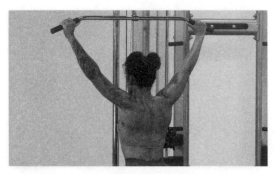 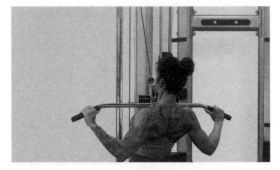

We're focusing here on your lats, one of the hardest muscles to engage. It's important to keep your chest lifted nice and high while leading the movement with your elbows.

Make sure to hold the bar with your palms facing away from you (pronated). Keep your shoulders away from your ears on the way up.

Lat V-Bar Pull-Down

BODY PART: Back
EQUIPMENT: Lat pull-down machine

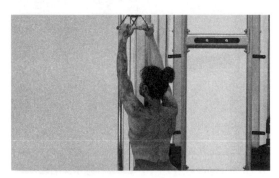 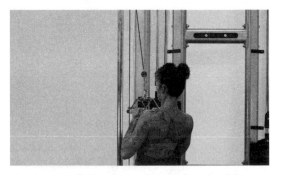

You're holding the V-bar for this one; make sure to retract your shoulder blades and don't let them elevate as you go up. Keep your chest up and core engaged.

As you pull the bar down, lead with your elbows and lean back slightly. Keep your shoulders away from your ears.

Lateral Jumping Jack

BODY PART: Full body (cardio)
EQUIPMENT: Bodyweight

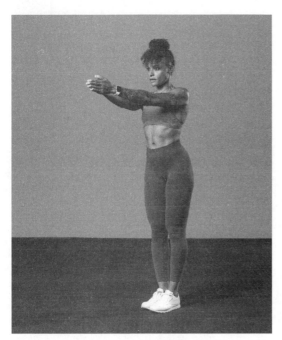 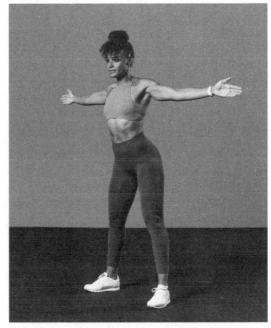

Keep your eyes looking straight ahead. Your arms and legs move together, your arms opening, horizontally aligned with the floor. Make sure to keep your shoulder blades contracted and your chest out the entire time—don't just swing your arms in and out.

Your goal is to control the movement and land smoothly and almost silently. Personally, I like to clap my hands every rep—it's like an auto high five!

Lateral Raise

BODY PART: Shoulders
EQUIPMENT: Dumbbells

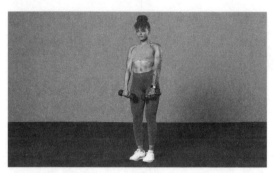 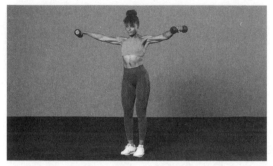

Bend your elbows slightly, keeping your chest up high and shoulders down, away from your ears.

Move your arms upward in a controlled fashion while keeping your shoulder blades retracted. Don't let the weights come slamming down; you want to move with control.

Leg Press

BODY PART: Legs
EQUIPMENT: Leg press

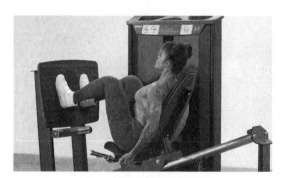 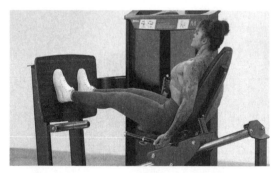

Set your feet about hip-width apart and your toes pointing slightly out. Even though you are seated, I want you to engage your core.

To get the most out of this exercise, bring your chest up nice and high. Be sure to keep your shoulders down and away from your ears.

Leg Press (Narrow Stance)

BODY PART: Legs
EQUIPMENT: Leg press

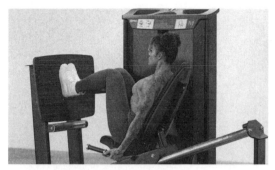

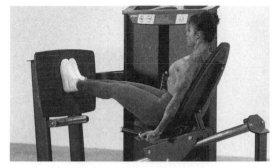

Set your feet closer than hip-width apart and your toes spread out inside your shoes. Keep your back pushed back against the chair. Move slowly and with control—no rush.

Do not lock your knees at the top of the movement.

Leg Press (Wide Stance)

BODY PART: Legs
EQUIPMENT: Leg press

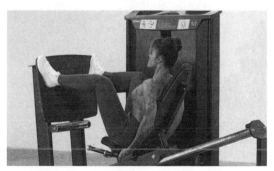

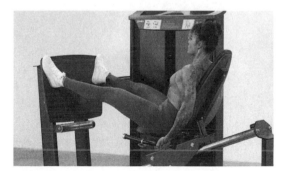

Separate your feet so they are at the edge of the platform. Make sure your toes are pointed outward and your knees are in line with your toes.

Bring your knees back as far as you can, and push through the heels on your way back, moving in a fluid motion.

LISS (Treadmill Walk)

BODY PART: Total body (cardio)
EQUIPMENT: Treadmill

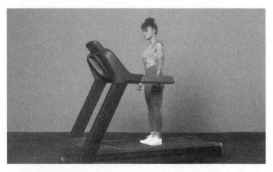
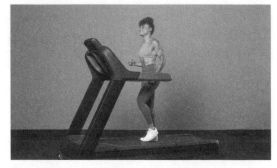

This is just like walking in the real world. Just make sure not to hold the rails of the treadmill unless it's needed.

Lunge, Alternating (Bodyweight)

BODY PART: Legs
EQUIPMENT: Bodyweight

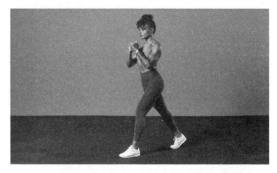
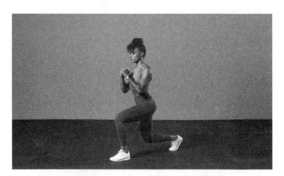

Focus on your form here. Push off your rear foot to stand up. Avoid leaning forward—just shoot upward in a straight line to stand. Keep your eyes looking forward.

Lying Leg Lift

BODY PART: Abs
EQUIPMENT: Bodyweight

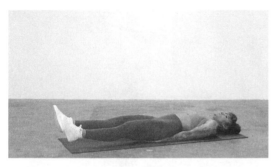 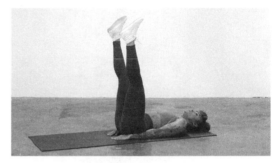

Push your lower back flat against the floor, lift your chest, slightly lift your feet off the ground, and then lift your legs to almost perpendicular with the floor, then back down.

The lower you get with your legs, the more it's going to work your core. Make sure you are looking straight up at the ceiling.

Lying Smith Machine Triceps Press

BODY PART: Triceps
EQUIPMENT: Smith machine

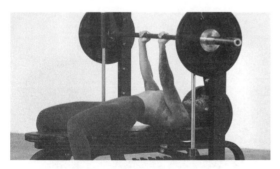 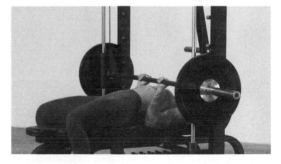

Using the Smith machine is really going to help with your form, so focus and get all your reps in with this exercise.

Take a narrow grip on the bar and keep your elbows tucked in tight toward your obliques. Press the bar with power and bring it back down with control in a smooth motion, exhale on the push, and inhale on your way down.

Military Press

BODY PART: Shoulders
EQUIPMENT: Barbell

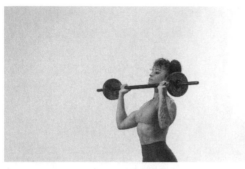

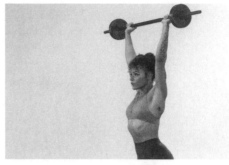

Keep your core engaged, and sit back into your hips to avoid overarching your back.

To get the most out of this exercise, don't go too far past your chin; this will keep your muscles engaged.

Mountain Climber

BODY PART: Full body (cardio)
EQUIPMENT: Bodyweight

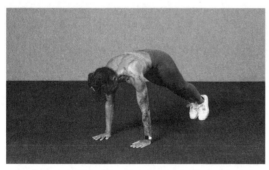

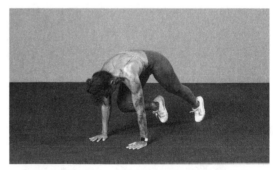

Start by getting into your plank (rounded upper back, butt tucked in, and abs contracted).

Keep your eyes looking straight at the floor and switch from right leg to left leg. Your feet should move about 12 inches back and forth as you switch. Maintain that plank!

Pec Deck

BODY PART: Chest
EQUIPMENT: Pec deck machine

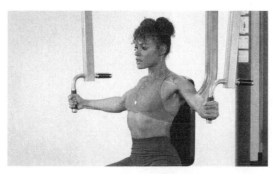

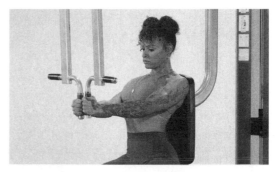

Sit tall with your core engaged. Your feet need to be planted flat in front of you.

You really want to think about squeezing your chest while keeping it up; don't let it cave in.

Plank Hold

BODY PART: Abs
EQUIPMENT: Bodyweight

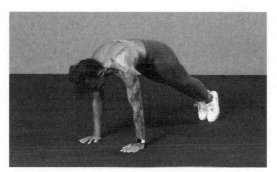

Get into a push-up position, round your upper back, tuck the butt in, and engage your abs. Be sure to squeeze your abs deeper as you exhale and inhale slowly.

Plyo Calf Raise

BODY PART: Legs
EQUIPMENT: Bodyweight

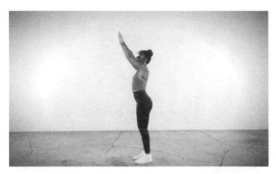 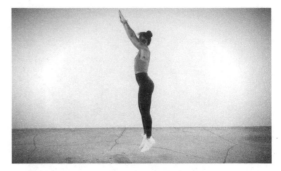

Jump off the front of your feet and don't let your heels touch the ground on the way down.

Reach your arms up high and tilt your chin up toward your hands.

Plyo Split Lunge

BODY PART: Legs
EQUIPMENT: Bodyweight

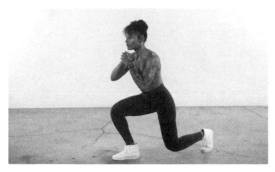 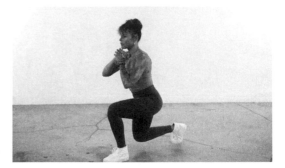

Keep your core tight and your hands in front of your chest. Push off your front foot and switch legs; remember to keep your hips square to avoid falling sideways.

Plyo Sumo

BODY PART: Legs
EQUIPMENT: Bodyweight

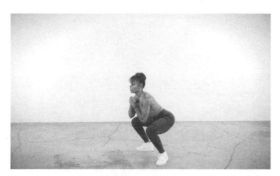 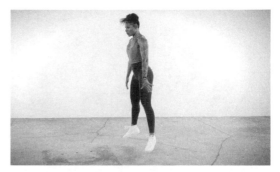

Keep your chest up and core tight. Your knees should remain in line with your toes. Push off your whole foot on the way up.

Pull-Up (Band Assisted)

BODY PART: Back
EQUIPMENT: Rack, band

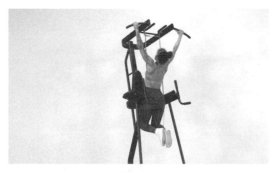 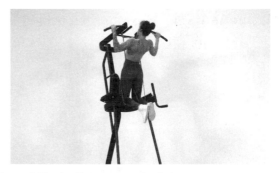

I know this exercise is challenging. Use a band that allows you to keep your reps smooth, and make sure you lift your chin up over the bar. (If you find you're not ready for a band, check to see if your gym has an assisted pull-up machine, which will provide a little more support until you're stronger.)

Lower all the way down while keeping your shoulder blades contracted.

Push-Up

BODY PART: Chest
EQUIPMENT: Bodyweight

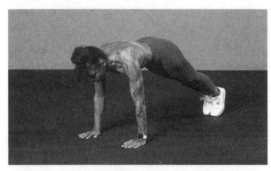

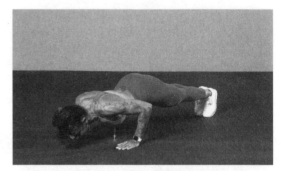

Assume a nice high plank with your upper back rounded slightly while your butt is tucked in (think booty to belly button connection).

Your hands should be slightly wider than shoulder-width apart, feet together. Inhale on the way down, exhale on the way up.

Quad Extension Machine

BODY PART: Legs
EQUIPMENT: Quad extension machine

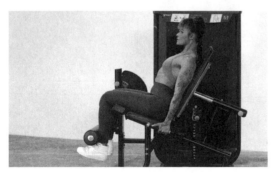

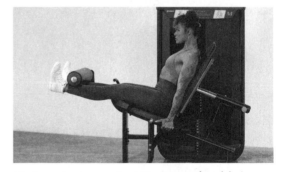

Sit tall in your seat, with your chest high to engage your core.

Make sure your booty is pushed into the seat really hard. Lift legs. Lower down with control.

Reverse Lunge (Dumbbells)

BODY PART: Legs
EQUIPMENT: Dumbbells

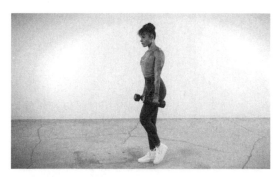 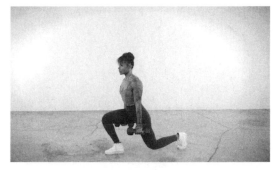

You want to create a 90-degree angle with your rear leg. If you feel a bit wobbly, check your core—your core and your grip on the weights should be tight.

Reverse Pec Deck

BODY PART: Back
EQUIPMENT: Pec deck machine

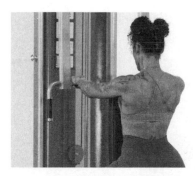 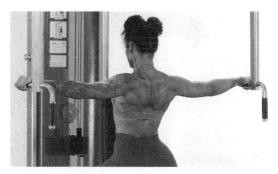

We're targeting the back of your shoulders here. Keep your spine tall, chest up, and wrists straight.

Every time you push the weight back, think of lifting your chest forward. Don't lose your form.

Reverse Pull-Up

BODY PART: Back
EQUIPMENT: Rack or Smith machine

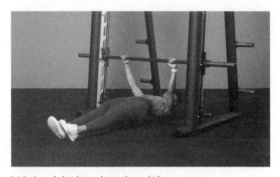 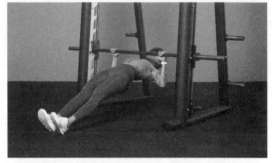

We're hitting back with power on this one. Set up the bar on the Smith machine or squat rack where you can grab it while being on the floor with arms fully extended.

Your job is to lift your entire body while keeping your back and legs aligned straight. Bring your chest to the bar every time.

Scissors

BODY PART: Abs
EQUIPMENT: Bodyweight

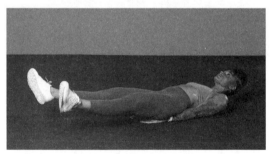 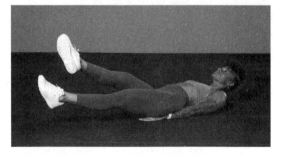

Sit on the floor or mat. Push your chest out and straighten your back. Lean back while keeping your back straight until your abs engage; place your arms under your butt with palms facing down.

Lift your legs and maintain position. Now proceed to scissor your legs left and right, alternating the top and bottom positions of each leg with every rep.

Seated Calf Raise

BODY PART: Legs
EQUIPMENT: Calf raise machine

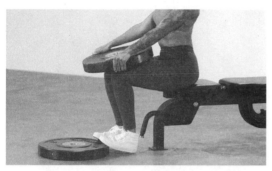 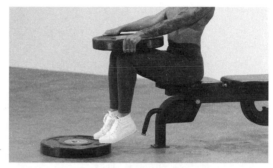

Choose a 25- to 45-lb. plate and place it on your knees. You can also use dumbbells. Place your heels slightly off the edge of medium-to-heavy plates.

Moving slowly, raise your heels high and squeeze your calves at the top. Then lower your heels and push them as far down as possible to get a full stretch.

Seated Shoulder Press

BODY PART: Shoulders
EQUIPMENT: Dumbbells

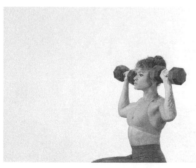 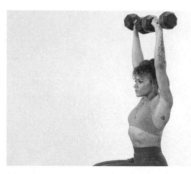

Keep your core engaged and sit back into your hips to avoid overarching your back. (Tuck your butt in and exhale into your abs.)

Keep your eyes looking forward. Be sure to exhale as you press up and inhale on the way down, controlling the movement and keeping your reps fluid.

Seated Smith Machine Shoulder Press

BODY PART: Shoulders
EQUIPMENT: Smith machine

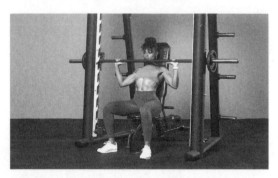

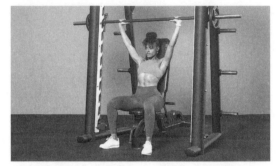

Keep your core engaged and sit back into your hips to avoid overarching your back. Tuck your butt in and squeeze your abs, keeping your chin tucked back and not down.

To get the most out of this exercise, don't go far past your chin—this will keep your muscles engaged and squeeze your shoulder blades at the top. Keep your reps fluid!

Seated Triceps Pull-Over

BODY PART: Triceps
EQUIPMENT: Dumbbell, bench

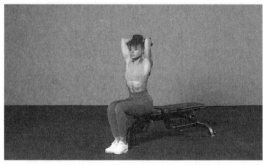

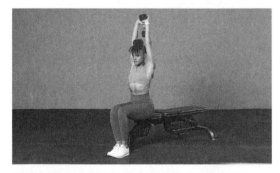

Sit down with your back completely straight, shoulder blades together, and chest out.

Hold the dumbbell between your thumb and index finger. Maintain elbows at 90 degrees, exhale and lift the dumbbell straight up; keep your elbows from flaring out.

Seated V-Bar Cable Row

BODY PART: Back
EQUIPMENT: Cable machine

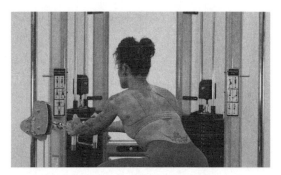 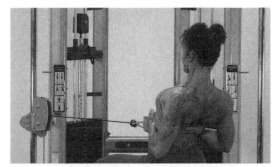

Lean forward as much as you can to start this move. When you pull back, lead with your elbows and let the bar touch your belly.

At the end of the move, lean back slightly and squeeze your shoulder blades, holding for a brief second before lowering the weight back. You can also use a row machine for this exercise.

Shoulder Press (Banded)

BODY PART: Shoulders
EQUIPMENT: Band

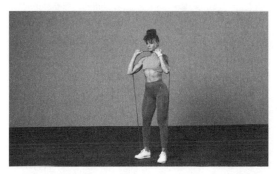 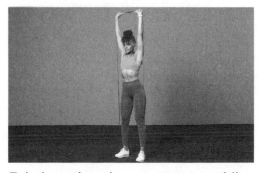

This is a killer shoulder exercise. Take a long band and make sure your chest is out and you're firmly stepping on the bottom part of the band.

Exhale and push your arms up while keeping your chin tucked back and shoulders retracted. Control the movement on the way down to about chin height and repeat.

Shoulder Press with Barbell

BODY PART: Shoulders
EQUIPMENT: Barbell

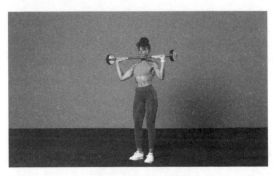

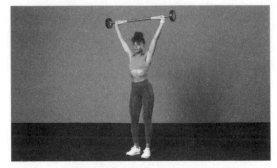

Keep your core engaged and sit back into your hips to avoid overarching your back.

To get the most out of this exercise, don't go far past your chin—this will keep your muscles engaged.

Shoulder Tap (in Plank Position)

BODY PART: Shoulders
EQUIPMENT: Bodyweight

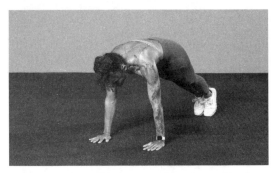

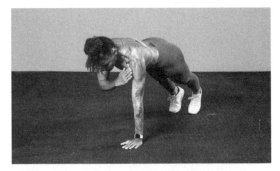

Assume the plank position (rounded upper back and butt tucked in).

With legs about hip-width apart, proceed to tap your left shoulder with your right hand, and vice versa. Be sure to exhale into your abs with every rep.

Single-Arm Dumbbell Press

BODY PART: Shoulders
EQUIPMENT: Dumbbells

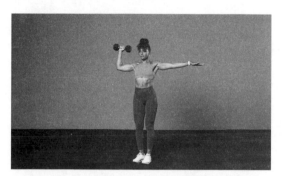

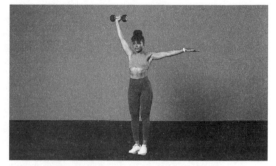

Keep your core engaged and sit back into your hips to avoid overarching your back. (Tuck your butt in and exhale into your abs.) Press the weight straight up and control it back to parallel with the floor.

Keep your eyes looking forward, and extend the opposite arm straight out, engaging your shoulder blades. Be sure to exhale on the way up and inhale on the way down; control the movement.

Single-Arm Dumbbell Row

BODY PART: Back
EQUIPMENT: Dumbbell, bench

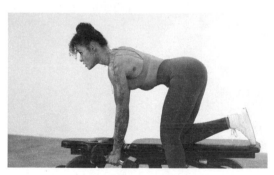

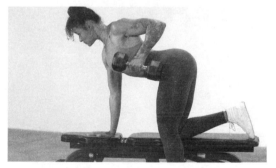

Drive your elbow up at the ceiling to initiate this movement.

Keep your chest locked in and think of pushing your chest forward every time you bring the weight to the side of your ribs.

Single-Leg Lying Hamstring Extension

BODY PART: Legs
EQUIPMENT: Hamstring extension machine

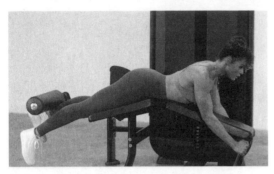

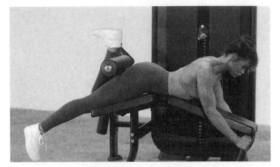

Think of a scooping motion as you bend your knee to bring your heel up to your butt, squeezing your hamstrings.

Play with the tempo on this one, 3 seconds on the way down, 1-second hold at the bottom, drive up with power (3,1,0 tempo).

Single-Leg Quad Extension

BODY PART: Legs
EQUIPMENT: Quad extension machine

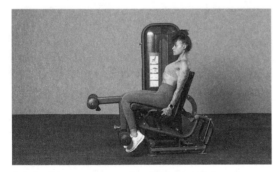

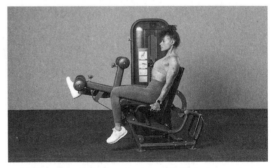

Sit tall in your seat with your chest high and booty pushed into the seat.

Play with the tempo on this one; try 3 seconds on the way down, 1-second hold at the bottom, drive up with power (3,1,0 tempo).

Skull Crusher (Incline Bench and Dumbbells)

BODY PART: Triceps
EQUIPMENT: Dumbbells, incline bench

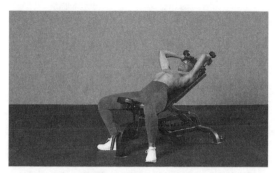

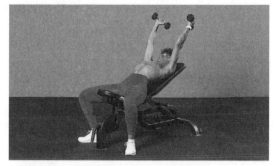

Keep your upper arms and elbows locked in. Hold the dumbbells between your thumbs and index fingers. Only your forearms should move in this exercise.

Make sure to lift toward the back of the room rather than up in order to keep the same angle as the bench. Keep your feet planted and butt stuck to the bench. Exhale on the work.

Skull Crusher (Incline Bench and E-Z bar)

BODY PART: Triceps
EQUIPMENT: E-Z bar, incline bench

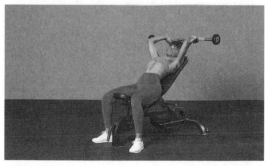

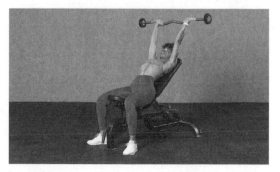

Keep your upper arms and elbows locked in. Only your forearms should move in this one.

Make sure to lift toward the back of the room rather than up in order to keep the same angle as the bench. Keep your feet planted and butt stuck to the bench. Exhale on the work.

Smith Machine Flat Chest Press

BODY PART: Chest
EQUIPMENT: Smith machine

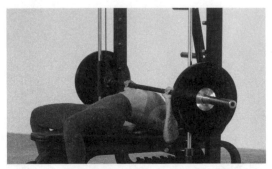 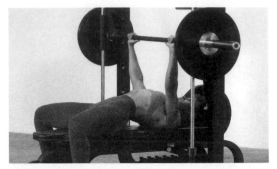

Take some time with this move. Focus on your form and pay attention to what it feels like to move the bar up and down.

Remember to breathe out on the way up and keep your chest locked in.

Smith Machine Front Squats

BODY PART: Legs
EQUIPMENT: Smith machine

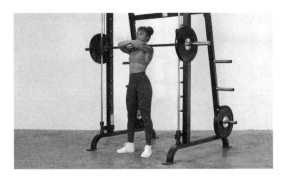 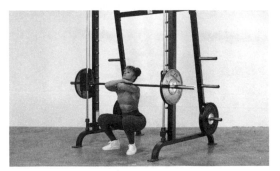

Rest the bar across your shoulders, and keep your shoulders and elbows aligned.

Sit low into your squat, a bit past 90 degrees. Squeeze your booty to push yourself up.

Sprint

BODY PART: Full body (cardio)
EQUIPMENT: Treadmill or turf

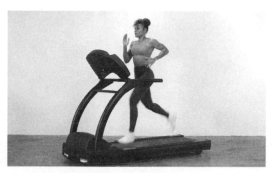

Alternate sprints with walking for the designated amount of time.

Pump your arms and use them to give you speed. Kick your heels up to your butt to get long strides. Run like you mean it!

Squat (Bodyweight)

BODY PART: Legs
EQUIPMENT: Bodyweight

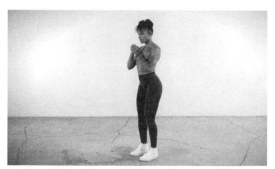
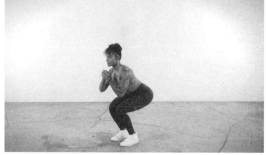

Place your feet about hip-width apart, hands in front of your chest. Keep your chest up nice and high, and your weight in your heels.

Get a bit lower than 90 degrees and really push yourself to work that booty, moving fluidly.

Squat (Wide Stance)

BODY PART: Legs
EQUIPMENT: Barbell

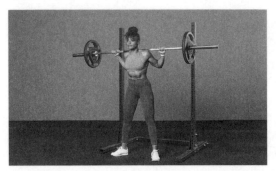 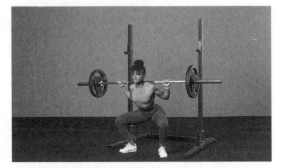

Keep your feet wider than hip-width apart, chest up, and hold the barbell right above your shoulder blades while keeping the wrists aligned with forearms.

Control the movement on the way down, then exhale and push up, focusing on your quads and hips. Make sure to come down to just past parallel with the floor.

Squat-Lunge-Squat-Lunge

BODY PART: Legs
EQUIPMENT: Bodyweight

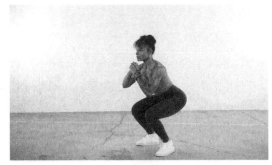 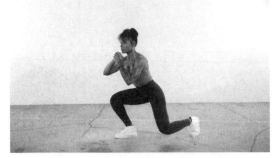

Start with your feet slightly wider than hip-width apart and move down as upright as possible while bringing your hips right below parallel with the ground.

Stay low and look straight ahead. Lunge backward with a strong 90-degree angle at the knee. Repeat squat and lunge with other leg.

Stairmaster

BODY PART: Full body (cardio)
EQUIPMENT: Stairmaster

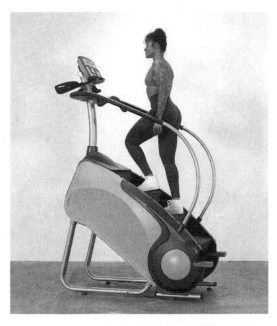

Set the stair climber at level 6.0. Remember to walk tall and avoid leaning forward. Push through your feet to straighten your leg before you lift the other.

This is really going to make you sweat! If you're looking for an extra challenge for your booty, perform 5 × 30 kick-backs, lifting from the heel.

Standing Calf Raise

BODY PART: Legs
EQUIPMENT: Calf raise or Smith machine

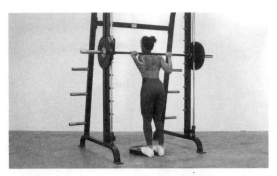 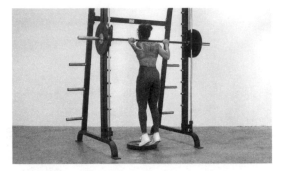

Hold the bar right on your trap muscles. Rise in a smooth motion and control your way back down.

Engage your core and slightly bend your knees the entire time. Lift your heels up as high as you can, squeezing as much as you can. Lower back down and move between reps in a fluid motion.

Standing Dumbbell Shoulder Press

BODY PART: Shoulders
EQUIPMENT: Dumbbells

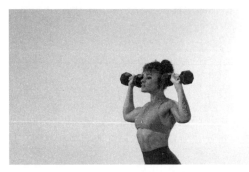 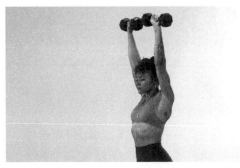

Keep your core engaged during this exercise and avoid overarching your back.

Exhale and press the dumbbells straight up. Squeeze your shoulders at the top and move the weights back down with control.

Standing Rope Triceps Pull-Over

BODY PART: Triceps
EQUIPMENT: Cable machine

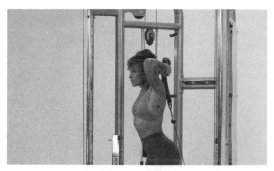

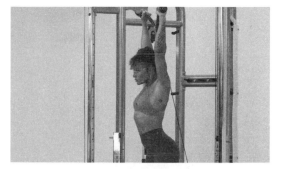

Keep your dominant foot forward; this is where most of your weight will be. In this exercise, you're facing away from the cable machine.

Keep your elbows aligned at about a 60-degree angle with the floor, exhale on the work, and keep the elbows stationary; only your forearms move.

Stationary Forward-Leaning Lunge with Dumbbells

BODY PART: Legs
EQUIPMENT: Dumbbells

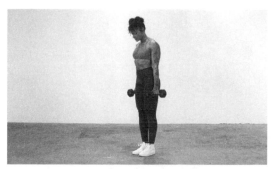

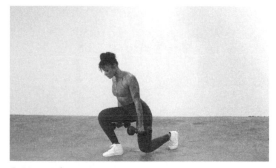

This exercise will test your balance. To maintain it, engage your core, keep your chest up, and squeeze all of your muscles.

Remember not to round your shoulders at the bottom.

Sumo Dead Lift

BODY PART: Legs
EQUIPMENT: Barbell

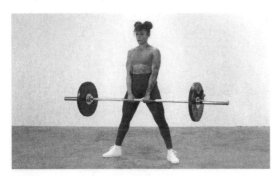

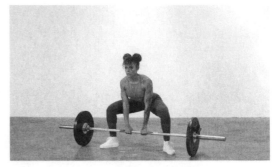

Anything sumo is going to work your inner thighs and booty. Keep your chest high as you push your hips back and down.

Your knees need to be in line with your toes the entire time. Think of squeezing your inner thighs together on your way up. Don't rush this move.

Sumo Squat

BODY PART: Legs
EQUIPMENT: Barbell

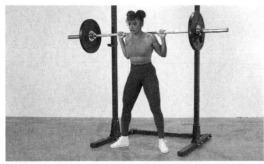

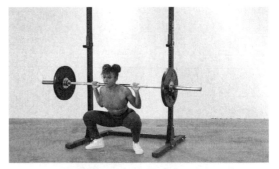

Focus on keeping the weight in your heels.

As you push back and drop into the squat, make sure your knees are in line with your toes the entire time.

Sumo Squat (Smith Machine)

BODY PART: Legs
EQUIPMENT: Smith machine

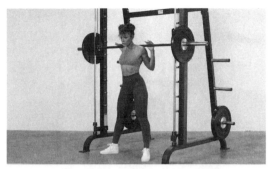

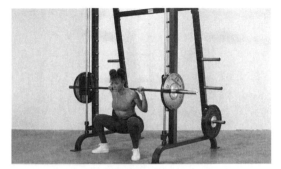

This is great for working your inner thighs and booty at the same time.

Keep your knees in line with your toes. Get low and engage your core.

Sumo Squat with Dumbbells

BODY PART: Legs
EQUIPMENT: Dumbbells

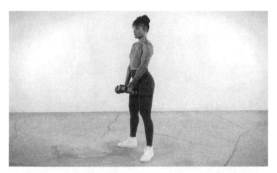

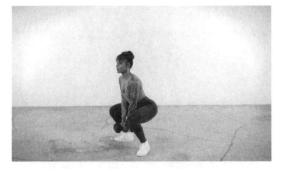

Keep your feet wider than hip-width apart and your chest up, and hold the dumbbells in front of you between your legs.

Control the movement on the way down, exhale, and push up, focusing on your quads and hips.

T-Bar Row

BODY PART: Back
EQUIPMENT: Barbell

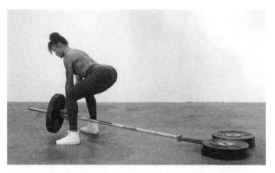

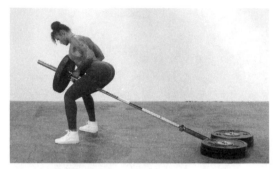

This is an awesome exercise that will target your lats and mid-back.

Concentrate on moving the weight with your back muscles by keeping your chest high. (This will allow you to avoid jerking the weight.)

Triceps Bent-Over Kick-Back

BODY PART: Triceps
EQUIPMENT: Dumbbells

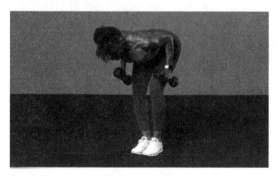

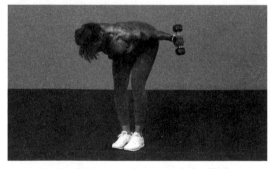

Start in a standing position and slowly bend at the hip until you're at about 60 degrees with the floor. Bend knees slightly.

Exhale and "kick" the dumbbells back while keeping the elbows parallel with the floor, moving smoothly.

Triceps Cable Pull-Down (Rope)

BODY PART: Triceps
EQUIPMENT: Cable machine

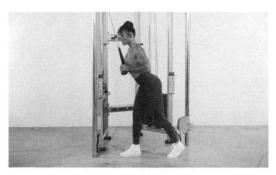

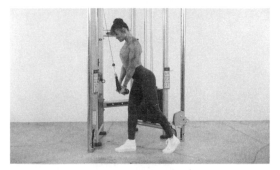

Keep your dominant foot forward; this is where most of your weight will be. Start with the rope at the same level as your diaphragm.

Keep your chest up to prevent your shoulders from caving in. Pull down rope.

Triceps Cable Push-Down (Straight Bar)

BODY PART: Triceps
EQUIPMENT: Cable machine

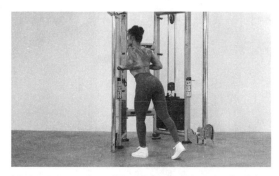

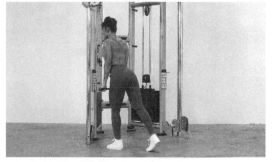

Keep your dominant foot forward; this is where most of your weight will be. Start with the bar right below your chest.

Exhale and push straight down while keeping your chest forward and wrists aligned with your forearms.

Triceps Dip Using Bodyweight (Bench)

BODY PART: Triceps
EQUIPMENT: Bench, bodyweight

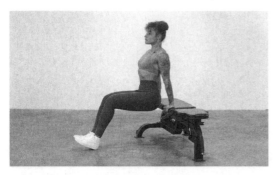 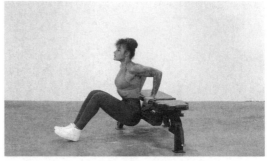

Align your wrists with your forearms while holding the edge of the bench. Your booty should be really close to the bench, with your chest high and shoulders pushed back. This will help avoid injury.

Focus on bending your arms at 90 degrees. Your elbows should not flare out; focus on pushing them inward the entire time.

Walk

BODY PART: Full body (cardio)
EQUIPMENT: Bodyweight

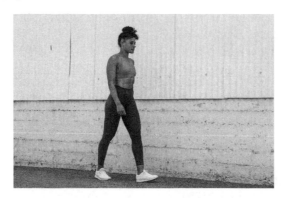

Walking Lunge (Bodyweight)

BODY PART: Legs
EQUIPMENT: Bodyweight

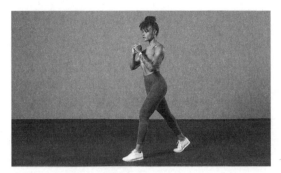 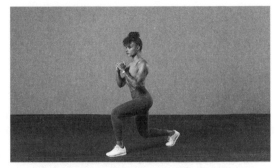

Focus on your form here. Step back and push off your rear foot to stand up, but don't lean forward; stand up in a straight line. Keep your eyes looking forward. Repeat with other leg.

Walking Lunge with Dumbbells

BODY PART: Legs
EQUIPMENT: Dumbbells

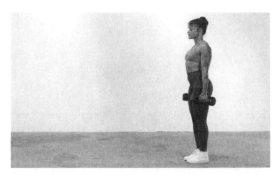 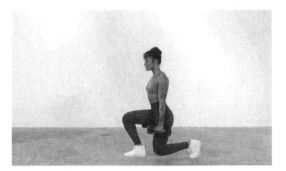

Step back slowly, taking two seconds on the way down, then pausing briefly at the bottom. Focus on getting low without your knee hitting the ground.

As you stand up, push up with your rear foot and go right into the next rep. Move with control by engaging your core.